Fibrinolytic Therapy in Clinical Practice

Fibrinolytic Therapy in Clinical Practice

Edited by

Freek Verheugt MD FESC FACC

Professor of Cardiology
Heartcenter, Department of Cardiology
University Medical Center St Radboud
6500 HB Nijmegen
The Netherlands

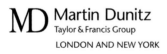
Martin Dunitz
Taylor & Francis Group
LONDON AND NEW YORK

© 2003 Martin Dunitz, an imprint of the Taylor & Francis Group plc

First published in the United Kingdom in 2003
by Martin Dunitz, an imprint of the Taylor & Francis Group plc
11 New Fetter Lane, London EC4P 4EE

Tel: +44 (0)20 7583 9855
Fax: +44 (0)20 7842 2298
E-mail: info@dunitz.co.uk
Website: http://www.dunitz.co.uk

Although every effort has been made to ensure that all owners of copyright material have been acknowledged in this publication, we would be glad to acknowledge in subsequent reprints or editions any omissions brought to our attention.

A CIP record for this book is available from the British Library.

ISBN 1 84184 081 5

Distributed in the USA by
Fulfilment Center
Taylor & Francis
10650 Toebben Drive
Independence, KY 41051 USA
Toll Free Tel: 1-800-634-7064
E-mail: taylorandfrancis@thomsonlearning.com

Distributed in Canada by
Taylor & Francis
74 Rolark Drive
Scarborough, Ontario M1R 4G2, Canada
Toll Free Tel: +1-877 226 2237
E-mail: tal_fran@istar.ca

Distributed in the rest of the world by
Thomson Publishing Services
Cheriton House, North Way
Andover, Hampshire SP10 5BE, UK
Tel: +44 (0)1264 332424
E-mail: salesorder.tandf@thomsonpublishingservices.co.uk

Composition by EXPO Holdings, Petaling Jaya, Malaysia

Printed and bound in Great Britain by Biddles Ltd. King's Lynn

Cover image shows the relationship between treatment delay and the absolute benefit per 100 treated patients (Fig. 2.5). Reproduced with kind permission from the Lancet.

Contents

List of contributors   vii

Preface   x

1. Pharmacology of thrombolytic agents   1
   H Roger Lijnen and Désiré Collen

2. General principles of fibrinolytic therapy in acute myocardial infarction
   Robert G Wilcox

3. Antiplatelet therapy   39
   Gianluca Gonzi, Silvia Buratti and Diego Ardissino

4. Anticoagulants as adjunctive therapy in fibrinolysis for acute myocardial infarction   63
   Marc A Brouwer and Freek W A Verheugt

5. Pharmacological interventions for acute myocardial infarction   75
   Preet Randhawa and William D Weaver

6. Percutaneous coronary intervention in acute ST–segment elevation of myocardial infarction   97
   Stephen G Ellis

7. Pre-hospital fibrinolytic therapy   111
   Eric Boersma

8. Fibrinolytic therapy in venous thromboembolism   131
   Marije ten Wolde, Maria M W Koopman and Harry R Büller

9. General principles of fibrinolytic therapy in ischaemic stroke   151
   Peter D Schellinger and Werner Hacke

Index   175

Contributors

Diego Ardissino
Professor and Chairman of the
Division of Cardiology
Heart Department
Maggiore Hospital
University of Parma
Italy

Eric Boersma
Thoraxcenter
Erasmus Medical Center
Dr Molewaterplein 40
3015 GD Rotterdam
The Netherlands

Marc A Brouwer
Heartcenter
540 Department of Cardiology
PO Box 9101
University Medical Center St
Radboud
6500 HB Nijmegen
The Netherlands

Harry R Büller
Academic Medical Center
Department of Vascular Medicine
Room F4-211, Meibergdreef 9
1105 AZ Amsterdam
The Netherlands

Silvia Buratti
Resident, Division of Cardiology
Heart Department
Maggiore Hospital
University of Parma
Italy

D Collen
Center for Molecular and Vascular
Biology
University of Leuven, Campus
Gasthuisberg, O&N
Herestraat 49, B-3000 Leuven
Belgium

Stephen G Ellis
Director, Sones Cardiac
Catheterization Laboratories
Department of Cardiology,
Desk F-25
Cleveland Clinic Foundation
9500 Euclid Avenue
Cleveland, OH 44195-0001
USA

Gianluca Gonzi
Clinical Assistant
Division of Cardiology
Heart Department
Maggiore Hospital
University of Parma
Italy

Werner Hacke
Neurologische Universitätsklinik
University of Heidelberg
Im Neuenheimer Feld 400
D-69120 Heidelberg
Germany

Maria M W Koopman
Academic Medical Center
Department of Vascular Medicine
Room F4-133, Meibergdreef 9
1105 AZ Amsterdam
The Netherlands

H Roger Lijnen
Center for Molecular and Vascular
Biology
University of Leuven, Campus
Gasthuisberg, O&N
Herestraat 49, B-3000 Leuven
Belgium

Preet Randhawa
Division of Cardiology
Henry Ford Heart and Vascular
Institute
2799 W. Grand Boulevard
Detroit, MI 482002
JSA

eter D Schellinger
urologische Universitätsklinik
L   iversity of Heidelberg
Ir   Neuenheimer Feld 400
D-   )120 Heidelberg
Ge   hany

Fre   W A Verheugt
Prof   sor of Cardiology
Hear   enter
540 C   )artment of Cardiology
PO Bc   9101
Univer   y Medical Center
St Rad.   ud
6500 H   Nijmegen
The Net.   rlands

William D Weaver
Division Head, Cardiology
Henry Ford Heart and Vascular
Institute
2799 W. Grand Boulevard
Detroit, MI 482002
USA

Robert G Wilcox
Department for Cardiovascular
Medicine
University Hospital
Nottingham NG7 2UH
UK

Marije ten Wolde
Academic Medical Center
Department of Vascular Medicine
Room F4-138, Meibergdreef 9
1105 AZ Amsterdam
The Netherlands

Preface

Fibrinolytic therapy of acute myocardial infarction has been the greatest breakthrough in the treatment of this most important cause of death in the Western world. Better angiographic knowledge of the pathogenesis of acute ST segment elevation coronary syndromes has identified acute vessel occlusion as the main mechanism. Thrombosis of the large arteries may have catastrophic consequences like sudden death, myocardial infarction, ischemic stroke and pulmonary embolism.

Early investigation of occluded blood vessels has been shown to improve symptoms, enhancing organ recovery and eventually improving quantity and quality of life.

There has been a dramatic evolution in drug design of fibrinolytic agents. Furthermore, adjuvant therapy has been introduced and evaluated in numerous clinical trials. Proper patient selection and evidence-based use of lytics and their adjunctive therapies form the mainstay of modern reperfusion therapy.

Fibrinolytic Therapy in Clinical Practice is a practical guideline in the clinical application of fibrinolytic therapy in a variety of life-threatening disorders. It is not an encyclopaedia of all trials, but shows the current guidelines for physicians taking care of acutely ill patients, whether in intensive units, coronary care units, ambulances or emergency departments.

Nijmegen, June 2003

Freek W.A. Verheugt, MD, FESC, FACC
Professor of Cardiology

1
Pharmacology of thrombolytic agents

H Roger Lijnen and Désiré Collen

Introduction

Thrombolysis consists of the pharmacological dissolution of a blood clot by intravenous infusion of plasminogen activators that activate the fibrinolytic system. The fibrinolytic system includes a proenzyme, plasminogen, which is converted by plasminogen activators to the active enzyme plasmin, which in turn digests fibrin to soluble degradation products. Inhibition of the fibrinolytic system occurs by plasminogen activator inhibitors (mainly plasminogen activator inhibitor-1, PAI-1) and by plasmin inhibitors (mainly α_2-antiplasmin) (Fig. 1.1). Thrombolytic agents that are either approved or under clinical investigation in patients with acute myocardial infarction include streptokinase, recombinant tissue-type plasminogen activator (rt-PA or alteplase), rt-PA derivatives, such as reteplase, lanoteplase and tenecteplase, anisoylated plasminogen-streptokinase activator complex (APSAC or anistreplase), two-chain urokinase-type plasminogen activator (tcu-PA or urokinase), recombinant single-chain u-PA (scu-PA or pro-urokinase, saruplase), and recombinant staphylokinase and derivatives. Fibrin-selective agents (rt-PA and derivatives, staphylokinase and derivatives and to a lesser extent scu-PA), which digest the clot in the absence of systemic plasminogen activation, are distinguished from non-fibrin-selective agents (streptokinase, tcu-PA and APSAC), which activate systemic and fibrin-bound plasminogen relatively indiscriminately (Fig. 1.1).[1,2] In this chapter, we will review the physicochemical properties, mechanism of action and pharmacodynamics of presently available thrombolytic agents.

Physicochemical properties of thrombolytic agents

t-PA and variants

Wild-type recombinant t-PA (alteplase, rt-PA) is a single-chain serine proteinase of 70 kDa, consisting of 527 amino acids with Ser as the NH_2-terminal amino acid; it was subsequently shown that native t-PA contains

Fluid phase

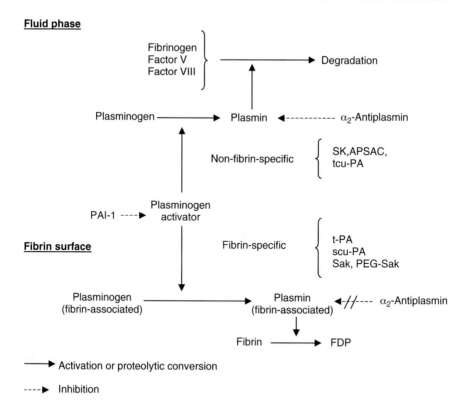

⟶ Activation or proteolytic conversion

----▶ Inhibition

Figure 1.1

In the fibrinolytic system, the proenzyme plasminogen is activated to the active enzyme plasmin by a plasminogen activator. Plasmin degrades fibrin into soluble fibrin degradation products (FDP). Inhibition may occur at the level of the plasminogen activator (inhibition of t-PA and u-PA by plasminogen activator inhibitor-1, PAI-1), or at the level of plasmin, mainly by α_2-antiplasmin. Non-fibrin-specific plasminogen activators (streptokinase, SK; anisoylated plasminogen streptokinase activator complex, APSAC; two-chain urokinase, tcu-PA) activate both plasminogen in the fluid phase and fibrin-associated plasminogen. Plasmin generated in the circulating blood is rapidly neutralized by α_2-antiplasmin, and excess plasmin may degrade other plasma proteins. Fibrin-specific plasminogen activators (tissue-type plasminogen activator, t-PA; single-chain u-PA, scu-PA; staphylokinase, Sak; pegylated Sak, PEG-Sak) preferentially activate fibrin-associated plasminogen. Fibrin-associated plasmin is protected from rapid inhibition by α_2-antiplasmin.

an NH$_2$-terminal extension of three amino acids, but in general the initial numbering system has been maintained. Limited plasmic hydrolysis of the Arg^{275}–Ile^{276} peptide bond converts t-PA to a two-chain molecule held together by one interchain disulphide bond. The t-PA molecule contains four domains: (1) an NH$_2$-terminal region of 47 residues (residues 4–50), which is homologous with the finger domains mediating the fibrin affinity of fibronectin; (2) residues 50–87, which are homologous with epidermal

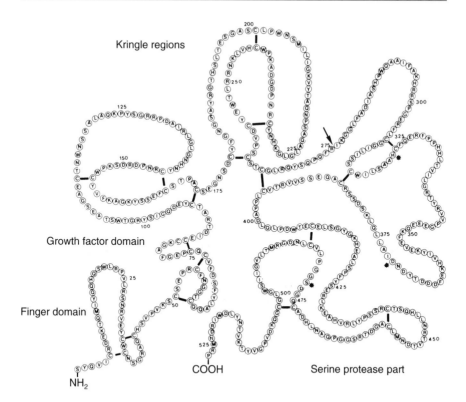

Figure 1.2

Schematic representation of the primary structure of t-PA. The amino acids are represented by their single letter symbols and black bars indicate disulphide bonds. The catalytic triad His[322], Asp[371] and Ser[478] is indicated with an asterisk. The arrow indicates the plasmin cleavage site for conversion of single-chain to two-chain t-PA.

growth factor; (3) two kringle regions comprising residues 87–176 and 176–262, which are homologous with the five kringles of plasminogen; and (4) a serine proteinase domain (residues 276–527) with the active site residues His[322], Asp[371] and Ser[478] (Fig. 1.2). The t-PA molecule comprises three potential *N*-glycosylation sites, at Asn[117], Asn[184] and Asn[448].[3] In contrast to the single-chain precursor form of most serine proteinases, single-chain t-PA is enzymatically active. Alteplase (rt-PA) is obtained by expression in Chinese hamster ovary cells.

By deletion or substitution of functional domains, by site-specific point mutations and/or by altering the carbohydrate composition, mutants of rt-PA have been produced with higher fibrin-specificity, more zymogenicity, slower clearance from the circulation and resistance to plasma proteinase inhibitors (Fig. 1.3).

Reteplase (Rapilysin[R] or Ecokinase[R]) is a single-chain non-glycosylated deletion variant consisting only of the kringle 2 and the proteinase domain

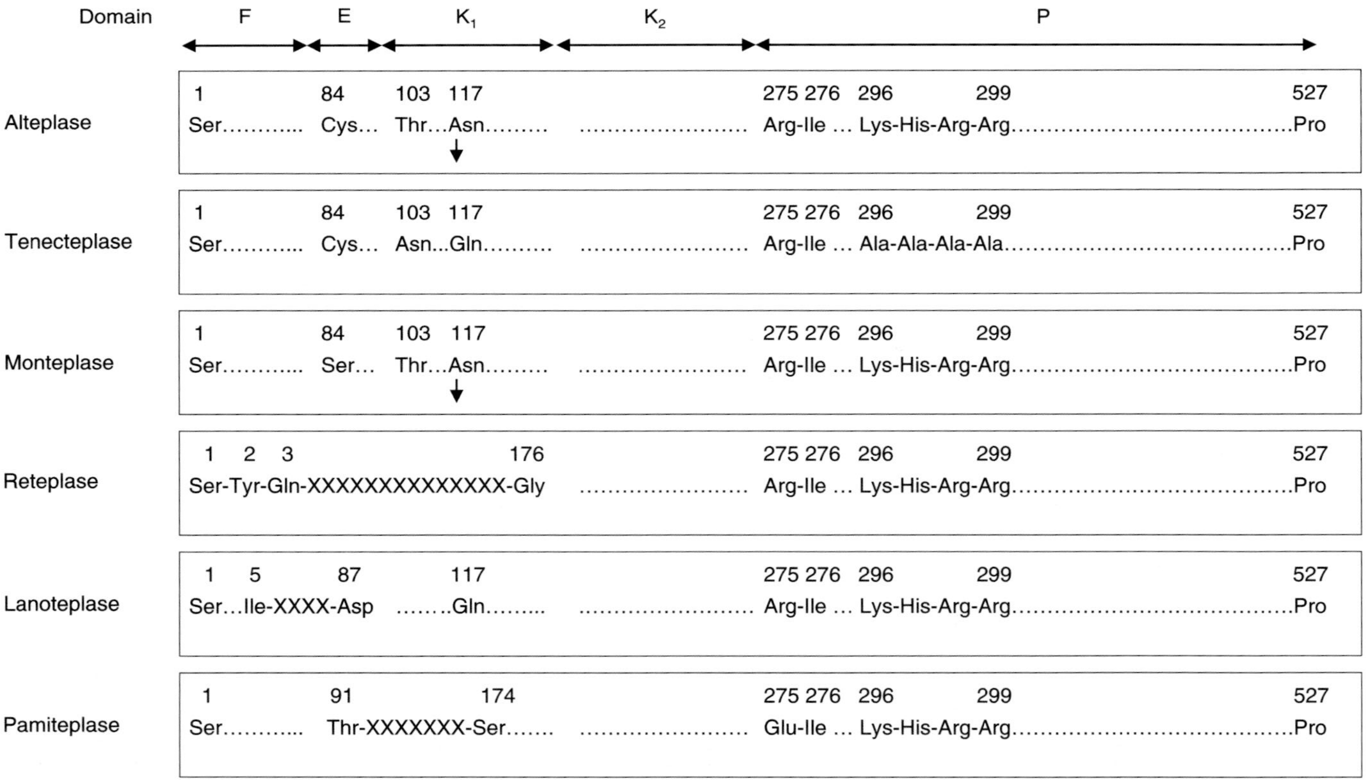

Figure 1.3

Schematic representation of the structure of wild-type t-PA (alteplase, rt-PA), tenecteplase, monteplase, reteplase, lanoteplase and pamiteplase. F, finger domain; E, growth factor domain; K_1 and K_2, kringle 1 and 2; P, proteinase domain; Asn, N-linked glycosylation; XXX, represents deleted sequences (for more details, see text).

of human t-PA; it contains amino acids 1–3 and 176–527 (deletion of Val^4–Glu^{175}); the Arg^{275}–Ile^{276} plasmin cleave site is maintained.[4]

In tenecteplase (TNK-rt-PA), replacement of Asn^{117} with Gln (N117Q) deletes the glycosylation site in kringle 1, whereas substitution of Thr^{103} by Asn (T103N) reintroduces a glycosylation site in kringle 1, but at a different locus; these modifications substantially decrease the plasma clearance rate. In addition, the amino acids Lys^{296}–His^{297}–Arg^{298}–Arg^{299} were each replaced with Ala, which confers resistance to inhibition by PAI-1.[5] Lanoteplase is a deletion mutant of rt-PA (without the finger and growth factor domains) in which glycosylation at Asn^{117} is lacking.[6] Monteplase has a single amino acid substitution in the growth factor domain (Cys^{84} to Ser),[7] and pamiteplase has deletion of the kringle 1 domain and substitution of Arg^{275} to Glu (rendering it resistant to conversion to a two-chain molecule by plasmin).[8]

Different molecular forms of the vampire bat (*Desmodus rotundus*) salivary plasminogen activator (DSPA) have been characterized. Two high M_r forms, DSPAα$_1$ (43 kDa) and DSPAα$_2$ (39 kDa) show about 85% homology with human t-PA, but contain neither a kringle 2 domain nor a plasmin-sensitive cleavage site. DSPAβ lacks the finger domain and DSPAγ lacks the finger and growth factor domains.[9]

u-PA moieties

Urokinase (u-PA) is secreted as a 54 kDa single-chain molecule (scu-PA, pro-urokinase) that can be converted to a two-chain form (tcu-PA). u-PA is a serine proteinase of 411 amino acids, with active site triad His^{204}, Asp^{255} and Ser^{356}. The molecule contains an NH$_2$-terminal growth factor domain and one kringle structure homologous to the kringles of plasminogen and t-PA.[10] u-PA contains only one *N*-glycosylation site (at Asn^{302}), and is fucosylated at Thr^{18}. Conversion of scu-PA to tcu-PA occurs after proteolytic cleavage at position Lys^{158}–Ile^{159} by plasmin, but also by kallikrein, trypsin, cathepsin B, human T-cell-associated serine proteinase-1 and thermolysin. A fully active tcu-PA derivative is obtained after additional proteolysis by plasmin at position Lys^{135}–Lys^{136}. Recombinant scu-PA (saruplase) has been expressed in *Escherichia coli* and is obtained as a 45 kDa nonglycosylated molecule.

Streptokinase and derivatives

Streptokinase is a non-enzyme protein produced by several strains of haemolytic streptococci. It consists of a single polypeptide chain of 47–50 kDa with 414 amino acids.[11] The region comprising amino acids 1–230 shows some homology with trypsin-like serine proteinases but lacks an active site serine residue.

APSAC (anistreplase, Eminase™) is an equimolar noncovalent complex between human lysine-plasminogen and streptokinase. The catalytic centre is located in the COOH-terminal region of plasminogen, whereas the lysine-binding sites (with weak fibrin affinity) are comprised within the NH_2-terminal region of the molecule. Specific acylation of the catalytic centre in the complex is achieved by the use of a reversible acylating agent, p-amidinophenyl-p'-anisate–HCl. This approach should prevent premature neutralization of the agent in the bloodstream and enable its activation to proceed in a controlled and sustained manner.[12]

Staphylokinase and derivatives

Staphylokinase (Sak) is a 135 amino acid protein (comprising 45 charged amino acids without cysteine residues or glycosylation), secreted by *Staphylococcus aureus* strains after lysogenic conversion or transformation with bacteriophages. The primary structure of Sak shows no homology with that of other plasminogen activators. Recombinant Sak is obtained by expression in *E. coli*.[13–15]

Staphylokinase folds into a compact ellipsoid structure in which the core of the protein is composed exclusively of hydrophobic amino acids. It is folded into a mixed five-stranded, slightly twisted β-sheet which wraps around a central α-helix and has two additional short two-stranded β-sheets opposing the central sheet.[16]

Wild-type Sak contains three immunodominant epitopes. A comprehensive site-directed mutagenesis programme resulted in the identification of variants with reduced antigenicity, but maintained fibrinolytic potency and fibrin-specificity, such as SakSTAR (K35A, E65Q, K74R, D82A, S84A, T90A, E99D, T101S, E108A, K109A, K130T, K135R) (code SY 155) and SakSTAR (K35A, E65Q, K74R, E80A, D82A, T90A, E99D, T101S, E108A, K109A, K130T, K135R) (code SY 161).[17] Furthermore, SY 161, with Ser in position 3 mutated into Cys, was derivatized with maleimide-substituted polyethylene glycol (P) with molecular weights of 5000 (P5), 10 000 (P10) or 20 000 (P20), and characterized *in vitro* and *in vivo* (cf. below).[18]

Mechanism of action of thrombolytic agents

t-PA and variants

t-PA is an ineffective enzyme in the absence of fibrin, but the presence of fibrin strikingly enhances the activation rate of plasminogen.[19] During fibrinolysis, fibrinogen and fibrin are continuously modified by cleavage with thrombin or plasmin, yielding a diversity of reaction products.[20] Optimal stimulation of t-PA is only obtained after early plasmin cleavage in the COOH-terminal Aα-chain and the NH_2-terminal Bβ-chain of fibrin, yielding fragment X-polymer. Kinetic data support a mechanism in which fibrin provides a surface to which t-PA and plasminogen adsorb in a sequential and ordered way, yielding a cyclic ternary complex.[19] Formation of this complex results in an enhanced affinity of t-PA for plasminogen, yielding up to three orders of magnitude higher catalytic efficiencies for plasminogen activation. This is mediated at least in part by COOH-terminal lysine residues generated by plasmin cleavage of fibrin. Plasmin formed at the fibrin surface has both its lysine binding sites and active site occupied and is thus only slowly inactivated by α_2-antiplasmin (half-life of about 10–100 s); in contrast, free plasmin, when formed, is rapidly inhibited by α_2-antiplasmin (half-life of about 0.1 s).[21] These molecular interactions mediate the fibrin specificity of t-PA.

Reteplase has a similar plasminogenolytic activity as wild-type rt-PA in the absence of a stimulator, but its activity in the presence of a stimulator is 4-fold lower, and its binding to fibrin is 5-fold lower. Reteplase and rt-PA are inhibited by PAI-1 to a similar degree.[4] Tenecteplase (TNK-rt-PA) has a similar ability as wild-type rt-PA to bind to fibrin, and lyses fibrin clots in a plasma milieu with enhanced fibrin specificity and delayed inhibition by PAI-1.[5] DSPAα1 and DSPAα2 exhibit a specific activity *in vitro* that is equal to or higher than that of rt-PA, a relative PAI-1 resistance and a greatly enhanced fibrin specificity with a strict requirement for polymeric fibrin as a cofactor.[9]

u-PA moieties

In contrast to tcu-PA, scu-PA displays very low activity toward low molecular weight chromogenic substrates, but it appears to have some intrinsic plasminogen-activating potential, which represents $\leq 0.5\%$ of the catalytic efficiency of tcu-PA.[22,23] In plasma, in the absence of fibrin, scu-PA is stable and does not activate plasminogen; however, in the presence of a fibrin clot, scu-PA, but not tcu-PA, induces fibrin-specific clot lysis.[22] scu-PA is an inefficient activator of plasminogen bound to internal lysine residues on intact fibrin, but has a higher activity toward plasminogen bound to newly generated COOH-terminal lysine residues on partially degraded fibrin.[24,25]

Streptokinase and derivatives

Streptokinase activates plasminogen indirectly, following a three-step mechanism.[26] In the first step, streptokinase forms an equimolar complex with plasminogen, which undergoes a conformational change resulting in the exposure of an active site in the plasminogen moiety. In the second step, this active site catalyses the activation of plasminogen to plasmin. In a third step, plasminogen-streptokinase molecules are converted to plasmin-streptokinase complexes. The active site residues in the plasmin-streptokinase complex are the same as those in the plasmin molecule. The main differences between the enzymatic properties of both moieties are that plasmin, in contrast to its complex with streptokinase, is unable to activate plasminogen, and is rapidly neutralized by α_2-antiplasmin, which does not inhibit the complex. Since streptokinase generates free circulating plasmin when α_2-antiplasmin becomes exhausted, its use is associated with generation of a systemic lytic state.

The reversible blocking of the catalytic site by acylation (APSAC) delays the formation of plasmin but has no influence on the lysine-binding sites involved in binding of the complex to fibrin, although the affinity of plasminogen for fibrin is very weak. Deacylation uncovers the catalytic centre, which converts plasminogen to plasmin.

Staphylokinase and derivatives

Sak forms a 1:1 stoichiometric complex with plasmin(ogen). It is not an enzyme, and generation of an active site in its equimolar complex with plasminogen requires conversion of plasminogen to plasmin. In plasma, in the absence of fibrin, no significant amounts of plasmin–Sak complex are generated because traces of plasmin are inhibited by α_2-antiplasmin. In the presence of fibrin, generation of the active complex is facilitated because traces of fibrin-bound plasmin are protected from α_2-antiplasmin, and inhibition of the complex by α_2-antiplasmin at the clot surface is delayed more than 100-fold. Furthermore, Sak does not bind to a significant extent to plasminogen in circulating plasma, but binds with high affinity to plasmin and to plasminogen which is bound to partially degraded fibrin.[27–29] During the activation process, the 10 NH_2-terminal amino acids of Sak are cleaved off. With SY 161-P5, this results in removal of the polyethylene glycol moiety.

Pharmacodynamics of thrombolytic agents

t-PA and variants

The initial and terminal half-lives of single-chain rt-PA, following infusion of 8.3 µg/kg/min over 30 min in healthy volunteers, were 3.3 min and 26 min.[30] In patients with acute myocardial infarction (AMI) clearance of single-chain rt-PA occurs with an initial half-life of 4–6 min.[31] Clearance is the result of interaction with several receptor systems. Liver endothelial cells have a mannose receptor that recognizes the high mannose-type carbohydrate side-chain at Asn^{117} in the kringle 1 domain, whereas liver parenchymal cells contain a calcium-dependent receptor which interacts mainly with the growth factor domain of t-PA.[32,33] In addition, the low-density lipoprotein receptor-related protein (LRP), expressed in high copy number on hepatocytes, binds free t-PA and complexes with PAI-1.[34,35]

The recommended dose of rt-PA (alteplase, Activase[R], Actilyse[R]) for the treatment of AMI was 100 mg administered as 60 mg in the first hour (of which 6–10 mg was a bolus over the first 1–2 min), 20 mg over the second hour, and 20 mg over the third hour. Later, it was proposed to give the same total dose of 100 mg but 'front loaded', starting with a bolus of 15 mg followed by 50 mg in the next 30 min and the remaining 35 mg in the following hour.[36] In the GUSTO trial, a dose of 15 mg intravenous bolus of alteplase followed by 0.75 mg/kg over 30 min (not to exceed 50 mg) and then 0.50 mg/kg over 60 min (not to exceed 35 mg) was utilized.[37] In the COBALT trial, double bolus administration of rt-PA (50 mg given 30 min apart) was evaluated in patients with myocardial infarction.[38] Whichever regimen is used, it is important to coadminister intravenous heparin during and after alteplase treatment. For catheter-directed local thrombolysis with alteplase in patients with recent peripheral arterial occlusion, a dose of 0.05–0.10 mg/kg per hour over an 8 hour period is used.

Mutants of rt-PA with higher fibrin specificity, more zymogenicity, slower clearance from the circulation and resistance to plasma proteinase inhibitors are presently under investigation at the preclinical level in animal models of venous and arterial thrombosis and in pilot studies, mainly in patients with AMI (Table 1.1).[2,39] During thrombolytic therapy there is a vast excess of t-PA over PAI-1 in the circulation, but critical lysis occurs at the surface of an arterial thrombus where the local PAI-1 concentration can be very high. Therefore, mutants with resistance to PAI-1 may be useful to reduce reocclusion. In addition, mutants with prolonged half-life may allow efficient thrombolysis by bolus administration at a reduced dose.

With reteplase, in patients an initial half-life of 14–18 min was observed. In the GUSTO-III trial, about 15 000 patients with acute myocardial infarction were randomly assigned to receive reteplase (2 boluses of 10 MU given 30 min apart) or 100 mg alteplase over 90 min. No clinical benefit of reteplase over alteplase could be demonstrated, in terms of 30 day mortality or frequency of haemorrhagic stroke, leading to the conclusion that both agents are equivalent.[40]

In patients with AMI, TNK-rt-PA (tenecteplase) has a half-life of 17 ± 7 min, as compared to 3.5 ± 1.4 min for rt-PA wild-type.[41] In the TIMI-10B trial, a phase II efficacy trial, a single bolus of 40 mg TNK-rt-PA yielded similar TIMI-3 flow rates at 90 min as accelerated rt-PA, with faster and more complete reperfusion.[42] In the ASSENT-2 study (about 17 000 patients with acute myocardial infarction of less than 6 h) 0.5 mg/kg bolus tenecteplase yielded similar 30 day mortality and rate of intracranial bleeding as front-loaded alteplase.[43]

With lanoteplase, given as a single bolus of 120 U/kg in the 'Intravenous n-PA for Treating Infarcting Myocardium Early (InTIME-II)' trial (about 15 000 patients), the 30 day mortality was similar to that

Table 1.1 Pharmacology of thrombolytic agents.

Agent	M_r (kDa)	Plasma $T_{1/2}$ (min)	Fibrin selectivity	Inhibition by PAI-1	Dose[a]	Antigenicity
Alteplase	70.0	4–8	++	Yes	100 mg/90 min	−
Tenecteplase	70.0	11–20	+++	No	≈ 0.5 mg/kg bolus	−
Reteplase	39.0	14–18	+	Yes	2 × 10 MU bolus, 30 min apart	−
Lanoteplase	53.5	23–27	+	Yes	120 MU/kg bolus	−
Monteplase	68.0	23	++	Yes	0.22 mg/kg bolus	−
Pamiteplase	58.0	30–47	++	Yes	0.1 mg/kg bolus	−
Saruplase	46.5	9	±	No	80 mg/60 min	−
Staphylokinase (Sak)	16.0	3–6	+++	No	20 mg/30 min	++
PEG-Sak	21.0	15	+++	No	5 mg bolus	+
Streptokinase	47–50	25[b]	−	No	1.5 × 10^6 U/60 min	++
APSAC	≈130.0	70[b]	±	No	30 U bolus[c]	++

[a] Most frequently used/tested dose in patients with acute myocardial infarction.
[b] Clearance half-life of the complex with plasminogen.
[c] 30 U APSAC contains about 1.1 × 10^6 U of streptokinase.

obtained with front-loaded alteplase, but the rate of intracerebral haemorrhage was significantly increased in the lanoteplase group.[44]

Monteplase has a half-life of 23 min following bolus injection of 0.22 mg/kg.[45] Pamiteplase has a half-life of 30–47 min following single bolus injection of 0.5–4 mg to human volunteers.[46] The latter two agents were investigated in dose-finding studies in patients with acute myocardial infarction,[47,48] but no large-scale trial on safety or mortality was reported.

In several animal models of thrombolysis DSPAα_1 has a 2.5 times higher potency and 4- to 8-fold slower clearance than rt-PA.[2,39] Patient data have not yet been reported.

u-PA moieties

The main mechanism of removal of u-PA from the blood is by hepatic clearance. scu-PA is taken up in the liver via a recognition site on parenchymal cells and is subsequently degraded in the lysosomes.[49] Following intravenous (i.v.) infusion of natural or recombinant scu-PA in patients with acute myocardial infarction, a biphasic disappearance was observed with initial half-lives in plasma (post-infusion) of 4 min or 8 min, respectively.[50,51]

With a preparation containing 160 000 IU/mg of saruplase, the dose used successfully in patients with acute myocardial infarction (PRIMI study) was 20 mg given as a bolus and 60 mg over the next 60 min, immediately followed by an i.v. heparin infusion (20 IU/kg per hour) for 72 h.[52] In the LIMITS study in patients with acute myocardial infarction, the same dose regimen of saruplase was used, but with a prethrombolytic heparin bolus of 5000 IU and an i.v. heparin infusion for 5 days starting 30 min after completion of thrombolysis.[53] A recombinant glycosylated form of pro-urokinase (A-74187) has been evaluated in patients with AMI using 60 mg or 80 mg monotherapy or 60 mg primed with a preceding bolus of 250 000 IU of recombinant tcu-PA, always combined with aspirin and i.v. heparin.[54]

Streptokinase and derivatives

The elimination half-life of streptokinase in man is approximately 20 min (initial half-life of 4 min and terminal half-life of 30 min).[55] In the last 15 years, high-dose (1.5 million units), short-term (15–60 min infusion) streptokinase treatment has been routinely used in patients with acute myocardial infarction. A few days after streptokinase administration, the antistreptokinase titre rises rapidly and remains high for at least 4–6 months, during which period renewed thrombolytic treatment with streptokinase or compounds containing streptokinase is impracticable since exceedingly high doses are required to overcome the antibodies.

The activity of APSAC is controlled by the deacylation rate; the deacylation half-life in human plasma is 105–120 min.[56] In healthy volunteers, an apparent clearance half-life of 70 min was found for anistreplase, as compared to 25 min for the plasminogen-streptokinase complex formed upon administration of streptokinase alone.[55] In patients with AMI treated with anistreplase, half-lives of 90–112 min were reported for the plasma clearance of fibrinolytic activity.[57]

The recommended dose of anistreplase in acute myocardial infarction is 30 U (1 mg = 1 U and 30 mg contains approximately 1.1×10^6 U of streptokinase) to be given as a bolus injection. In aggregate, comparative studies indicate that the efficacy for coronary thrombolysis of anistreplase is comparable or somewhat higher than i.v. streptokinase but lower than intracoronary streptokinase.[58] Since anistreplase contains streptokinase, it causes immunization. The antibody titre may increase up to 60-fold within 2–3 weeks and still be very high after 3 months.[59,60]

Staphylokinase and derivatives

In patients with AMI treated with an i.v. infusion of 10 mg staphylokinase (SakSTAR) over 30 min, the concentration of staphylokinase-related antigen in blood at the end of the infusion increased to between 0.9 μg/ml and 1.7 μg/ml. The post-infusion disappearance of staphylokinase-related antigen from plasma occurred in a biphasic manner with a $T_{1/2\alpha}$ of 6.3 min and a $T_{1/2\beta}$ of 37 min, corresponding to a plasma clearance of 270 ml/min.[61] In the STAR trial, SakSTAR antigen levels in 25 patients with acute myocardial infarction receiving 10 mg i.v. over 30 min were 0.56 ± 0.06 μg/ml at 25 min and 0.16 ± 0.04 μg/ml at 90 min, with corresponding levels of 1.9 ± 0.22 μg/ml and 0.42 ± 0.06 μg/ml in 23 patients receiving 20 mg SakSTAR over 30 min.[62]

Intravenous staphylokinase (10 mg or 20 mg), combined with heparin and aspirin, was shown to be a potent, rapidly acting and highly fibrin-selective thrombolytic agent in patients with AMI.[27–29] The CAPTORS trial (Collaborative Angiographic Patency Trial Of Recombinant Staphylokinase) studied the optimal dose of Sak required to achieve TIMI perfusion grade 3 flow at 90 min within an acceptable safety profile.[63] In this open-label angiographically controlled, dose-finding study, patients (≤ 80 years) with an AMI within 6 hours of symptom onset received Sak (Sak42D) as a bolus (20% of total dose) followed by an i.v. infusion over a 30 min period. Three incremental doses of Sak were studied: 15 mg (n = 21), 30 mg (n = 31) and 45 mg (n = 30). Surprisingly, there was no difference in TIMI-3 patency rates between the three doses given (62%, 65% and 63%, respectively). Four patients had a major bleeding, nine had a minor bleeding, but no patients had intracranial haemorrhage. There was no relation between the dose of Sak and the extent of bleeding. No patients experienced allergic reactions.

A second multicentre randomized trial compared the effects of double bolus Sak administration versus the accelerated and weight-adjusted rt-PA, on early coronary artery patency in 102 patients with AMI.[64] Patients randomized to double bolus Sak ($n = 50$) were given 15 mg over 5 min, with a second bolus of 15 mg 30 min later—68% of the patients receiving double bolus Sak had a TIMI-3 flow after 90 min versus 57% after rt-PA administration (RR 1.3; 95% CI 0.8–2.0, $p = 0.3$). At 24 hours, TIMI-3 rates were 100% in the Sak group, and 79% in the t-PA-treated group ($p = 0.005$). This difference at 24 hours is possibly related to the low procoagulant and proaggregatory side-effects of Sak.[65] The rates of haemorrhagic, mechanical and electrical complications did not significantly differ between treatment groups. Double bolus administration of Sak also preserved plasma fibrinogen and plasminogen levels, while α_2-antiplasmin levels had marginally but significantly decreased (91% of pretreatment values). In contrast, rt-PA caused a significant drop of fibrinogen (mean decrease versus pretreatment of 30% at 90 min) and of plasminogen and α_2-antiplasmin (mean decreases of 54% and 56%, respectively at 90 min).

However, most patients develop high titres of neutralizing specific immunoglobulin G (IgG) after infusion of staphylokinase, which would predict therapeutic refractoriness upon repeated administration. Efforts have been undertaken to reduce the immunogenicity of staphylokinase by site-directed mutagenesis and to reduce the plasma clearance by derivation with polyethylene glycol (PEG).

Thus, a recombinant Sak variant with reduced immunogenicity (SY 161) in which Ser in position 3 of the protein sequence was mutated into Cys, Sak (S3C, K35A, E65Q, K74R, E80A, D82A, T90A, E99D, T101S, E108A, K109A, K130T, K135R) was derivatized with maleimide-substituted PEG (P) with molecular weights of 5000 (P5), 10 000 (P10) or 20 000 (P20).[18] SakSTAR-related antigen following bolus injection disappeared from plasma with an initial half-life of 13, 30 and 120 min and was cleared at a rate of 75, 43 and 8 ml/min for variants substituted with P5, P10 and P20, respectively, as compared to an initial half-life of 3 min and a clearance of 360 ml/min for wild-type staphylokinase.[18] Intravenous bolus injection of 5 mg of the P5 variant in 18 patients with acute myocardial infarction restored TIMI-3 flow at 60 min in 14 patients. On the basis of these results, the staphylokinase mutant SY 161 substituted with a single PEG molecule with a molecular weight of 5000, has been selected for clinical development as a single i.v. bolus agent for thrombolytic therapy of AMI.

Conclusions

Presently available thrombolytic agents include non-fibrin-specific plasminogen activators (streptokinase, tcu-PA, APSAC) and fibrin-specific agents (t-PA, scu-PA, staphylokinase). The clinical benefits of thrombolytic therapy in patients with acute myocardial infarction are well documented, and a close correlation between early coronary artery recanalization and clinical outcome is established. However, all available thrombolytic agents still have significant shortcomings, including the need for large therapeutic doses, limited fibrin specificity and significant associated bleeding tendency and reocclusion. As a promising new development towards improvement of thrombolytic agents, mutants and variants of tissue-type plasminogen activator have been produced with reduced plasma clearance and lower reactivity with proteinase inhibitors and with maintained or enhanced plasminogen activator potency and/or fibrin specificity. In addition, the bacterial plasminogen activator staphyloki-nase has shown promise for fibrin-specific thrombolysis, although neutral-izing antibodies are elicited in most patients. Pegylated staphylokinase variants have been produced with reduced immunogenicity and pro-longed circulating half-life. The potential therapeutic benefit of these new agents is presently evaluated in large-scale randomized efficacy and safety studies in patients with thromboembolic diseases.

References

1. Collen D. Thrombolytic therapy. Thromb Haemost 1997; **78**:742–6.

2. Lijnen HR, Collen D. Tissue-type plasminogen activator. In: Barrett AJ, Rawlings ND, Woessner JF, eds, Handbook of proteolytic enzymes (Academic Press: London, 1998) 184–90.

3. Pennica D, Holmes WE, Kohr WJ et al. Cloning and expression of human tissue-type plasminogen activator cDNA in *E. coli*. Nature 1983; **301**:214–21.

4. Kohnert U, Rudolph R, Verheijen JH et al. Biochemical properties of the kringle 2 and protease domains are maintained in the refolded t-PA deletion variant BM 06.022. Prot Engineer 1992; **5**:93–100.

5. Paoni NF, Keyt BA, Refino CJ et al. A slow clearing, fibrin-specific, PAI-1 resistant variant of t-PA (T103N, KHRR296–299AAAA). Thromb Haemost 1993; **70**:307–12.

6. Den Heijer P, Vermeer F, Ambrosioni E et al. Evaluation of a weight-adjusted single-bolus plasminogen activator in patients with myocardial infarction: a double-blind, randomized angio-graphic trial of lanoteplase ver-sus alteplase. Circulation 1998; **98**:2117–25.

7. Suzuki S, Saito M, Suzuki N et al. Thrombolytic properties of a novel modified human tissue-type plasminogen activator (E6010): a bolus injection of E6010 has equivalent potency of lysing young and aged canine coronary thrombi. J Cardiovasc Pharmacol 1991; **17**:738–46.

8. Katoh M, Suzuki Y, Miyamoto T et al. Biochemical and pharmaco-kinetic properties of YM866, a novel fibrinolytic agent. Thromb Haemost 1991; **65**:1193 (Abstract 1794).

9. Krätzschmar J, Haendler B, Langer G. The plasminogen activator family from the salivary gland of the vampire bat *Desmodus rotundus*: cloning

and expression. Gene 1991; **105**:229–37.

10. Holmes WE, Pennica D, Blaber M et al. Cloning and expression of the gene for pro-urokinase in *Escherichia coli.* Biotechnology 1985; **3**:923–9.

11. Jackson KW, Tang J. Complete amino acid sequence of streptokinase and its homology with serine proteases. Biochemistry 1982; **21**:6620–5.

12. Smith RAG, Dupe RJ, English PD, Green J. Fibrinolysis with acyl-enzymes: a new approach to thrombolytic therapy. Nature 1981; **290**:505–8.

13. Sako T, Tsuchida N. Nucleotide sequence of the staphylokinase gene from *Staphylococcus aureus.* Nucleic Acids Res 1983; **11**:7679–93.

14. Behnke D, Gerlach D. Cloning and expression in *Escherichia coli, Bacillus subtilis* and *Streptococcus sanguis* of a gene for staphylokinase: a bacterial plasminogen activator. Mol Gen Genet 1987; **210**:528–34.

15. Collen D, Zhao ZA, Holvoet P, Marynen P. Primary structure and gene structure of staphylokinase. Fibrinolysis 1992; **6**:226–31.

16. Rabijns A, De Bondt HL, De Ranter C. Three-dimensional structure of staphylokinase, a plasminogen activator with therapeutic potential. Nat Struct Biol 1997; **4**:357–60.

17. Laroche Y, Heymans S, Capaert S, De Cock F, Demarsin E, Collen D. Recombinant staphylokinase variants with reduced antigenicity due to elimination of B-lymphocyte epitopes. Blood 2000; **96**:1425–32.

18. Collen D, Sinnaeve P, Demarsin E et al. Polyethylene glycol-derivatized cysteine-substitution variants of recombinant staphylokinase for single-bolus treatment of acute myocardial infarction. Circulation 2000; **102**:1766–72.

19. Hoylaerts M, Rijken DC, Lijnen HR et al. Kinetics of the activation of plasminogen by human tissue plasminogen activator. Role of fibrin. J Biol Chem 1982; **257**:2912–19.

20. Thorsen S. The mechanism of plasminogen activation and the variability of the fibrin effector during tissue-type plasminogen activator-mediated fibrinolysis. Ann NY Acad Sci 1992; **667**:52–63.

21. Collen D. On the regulation and control of fibrinolysis. Thromb Haemost 1980; **43**:77–89.

22. Gurewich V, Pannell R, Louie S et al. Effective and fibrin-specific clot lysis by a zymogen precursor form of urokinase (pro-urokinase). A study in vitro and in two animal species. J Clin Invest 1984; **73**:1731–9.

23. Lijnen HR, Van Hoef B, Nelles L, Collen D. Plasminogen activation with single-chain urokinase-type plasminogen activator (scu-PA). Studies with active site mutagenized plasminogen (Ser740 $\longrightarrow$ Ala) and plasmin-resistant scu-PA (Lys158 $\longrightarrow$ Glu). J Biol Chem 1990; **265**:5232–6.

24. Liu JN, Gurewich V. Fragment E-2 from fibrin substantially enhances pro-urokinase-induced Glu-plasminogen activation. A kinetic study using the plasmin-resistant mutant pro-urokinase Ala-158-rpro-UK. Biochemistry 1992; **31**:6311–17.

25. Fleury V, Lijnen HR, Anglès-Cano E. Mechanism of the enhanced intrinsic activity of single-chain urokinase-type plasminogen activator during ongoing fibrinolysis. J Biol Chem 1993; **268**:18554–9.

26. Reddy KNN. Mechanism of activation of human plasminogen by streptokinase. In: Kline DL, Reddy KNN, eds, Fibrinolysis

(CRC Press: Boca Raton, FL, 1980) 71–94.

27. Lijnen HR, Collen D. Staphylokinase, a fibrin-specific bacterial plasminogen activator. Fibrinolysis 1996; **10**:119–26.

28. Collen D. Staphylokinase: a potent, uniquely fibrin-selective thrombolytic agent. Nat Med 1998; **4**:279–84.

29. Collen D. The plasminogen (fibrinolytic) system. Thromb Haemost 1999; **82**:259–70.

30. Seifried E, Tanswell P, Rijken DC et al. Pharmacokinetics of antigen and activity of recombinant tissue-type plasminogen activator after infusion in healthy volunteers.Artzneimittel-Forschung 1988; **38**:418–22.

31. Garabedian HD, Gold HK, Leinbach RC et al. Comparative properties of two clinical preparations of recombinant human tissue-type plasminogen activator in patients with acute myocardial infarction. J Am Coll Cardiol 1987; **9**:599–607.

32. Otter M, Zockova P, Kuiper J, van Berkel TJ, Barrett-Bergshoeff MM, Rijken DC. Isolation and characterization of the mannose receptor from human liver potentially involved in the plasma clearance of tissue-type plasminogen activator. Hepatology 1992; **16**:54–9.

33. Kuiper J, Van't Hof A, Otter M, Biessen EAL, Rijken DC, van Berkel ThJC. Interaction of mutants of tissue-type plasminogen activator with liver cells: effect of domain deletions. Biochem J 1996; **313**:775–80.

34. Orth K, Madison EL, Gething MJ, Sambrook JF, Herz J. Complexes of tissue-type plasminogen activator and its serpin inhibitor plasminogen-activator inhibitor type 1 are internalized by means of the low density lipoprotein receptor-related protein/alpha 2-macroglobulin receptor. Proc Natl Acad Sci USA 1992; **89**:7422–6.

35. Bu G, Williams S, Strickland DK, Schwartz AL. Low density lipoprotein receptor-related protein/ alpha 2-macroglobulin receptor is an hepatic receptor for tissue-type plasminogen activator. Proc Natl Acad Sci USA 1992; **89**:7427–31.

36. Neuhaus KL, Feuerer W, Jeep-Tebbe S, Niederer W, Vogt A, Tebbe U. Improved thrombolysis with a modified dose regimen of recombinant tissue-type plasminogen activator. J Am Coll Cardiol 1989; **14**:1566–9.

37. GUSTO investigators. An international randomized trial comparing four thrombolytic strategies for acute myocardial infarction. N Engl J Med 1993; **329**:673–82.

38. COBALT investigators. A comparison of continuous infusion of alteplase with double-bolus administration for acute myocardial infarction. N Engl J Med 1997; **337**:1124–30.

39. Lijnen HR, Collen D. Strategies for the improvement of thrombolytic agents. Thromb Haemost 1991; **66**:88–110.

40. GUSTO-III investigators. A comparison of reteplase with alteplase for acute myocardial infarction. N Engl J Med 1997; **337**:1118–23.

41. Cannon CP, McCabe CH, Gibson CM et al. TNK-tissue plasminogen activator in acute myocardial infarction: results of the Thrombolysis in Myocardial Infarction (TIMI) 10A dose-ranging trial. Circulation 1997; **95**:351–6.

42. Cannon CP, Gibson MC, McCabe CH et al. TNK-tissue plasminogen

activator compared with front-loaded tissue plasminogen activator in acute myocardial infarction: results of the TIMI-10B trial. Circulation 1998; **98**:2805–14.

43. Assessment of the Safety and Efficacy of a New Thrombolytic (ASSENT-2) investigators. Single-bolus tenecteplase compared with front-loaded alteplase in acute myocardial infarction: the ASSENT-2 double-blind randomised trial. Lancet 1999; **354**:716–22.

44. Antman EM, Wilcox RG, Giugliano RP et al. Long term comparison of lanoteplase and alteplase in ST elevation myocardial infarction: 6 month follow-up in InTime-II trial. Circulation 1999; **100**:498 (Abstract).

45. Kawai C, Hosada S, Kimata S et al. Coronary thrombolysis in acute myocardial infarction of E6010 (novel modified t-PA): a multicenter, double-blind dose-finding study. Jpn Pharmacol Ther 1994; **22**:3925–50.

46. Hashimoto K, Oikawa K, Miyamoto I et al. Phase I study of a novel modified t-PA. Jpn J Med Pharm Sci 1996; **36**:623–46.

47. Kawai C, Yui Y, Hosada S et al. A prospective, randomized, double-blind multicenter trial of a single bolus injection of the novel modified t-PA E6010 in the treatment of acute myocardial infarction: comparison with native t-PA. J Am Coll Cardiol 1997; **29**:1447–53.

48. Yui Y, Haze K, Kawai C et al. Randomized, double-blind multi-center trial of YM866 (modified t-PA) by intravenous bolus injection in patients with acute myocardial infarction in comparison with tisokinase (native t-PA). J New Remedies Clin 1996; **45**:2175–221.

49. Kuiper J, Rijken DC, de Munk GAW, van Berkel TJ. In vivo and in vitro interaction of high and low molecular weight single-chain urokinase-type plasminogen activator with rat liver cells. J Biol Chem 1992; **267**:1589–95.

50. Van de Werf F, Nobuhara M, Collen D. Coronary thrombolysis with human single chain urokinase-type plasminogen activator (scu-PA) in patients with acute myocardial infarction. Ann Intern Med 1986; **104**:345–8.

51. Van de Werf F, Vanhaecke J, De Geest H, Verstraete M, Collen D. Coronary thrombolysis with recombinant single-chain urokinase-type plasminogen activator (rscu-PA) in patients with acute myocardial infarction. Circulation 1986; **74**:1066–70.

52. PRIMI Trial Study Group. Randomised double-blind trial of recombinant pro-urokinase against streptokinase in acute myocardial infarction. Lancet 1989; **1**:863–8.

53. Tebbe U, Windeler J, Boesl I et al on behalf of the LIMITS Study Group. Thrombolysis with recombinant unglycosylated single-chain urokinase-type plasminogen activator (Saruplase) in acute myocardial infarction: influence on early patency rate (LIMITS Study). J Am Coll Cardiol 1995; **26**:365–73.

54. Weaver WD, Hartmann JR, Anderson JL, Reddy PS, Sobolski JC, Sasahara AA for the Prourokinase Study Group. New recombinant glycosylated prourokinase for treatment of patients with acute myocardial infarction. J Am Coll Cardiol 1994; **24**:1242–8.

55. Staniforth DH, Smith RAG, Hibbs M. Streptokinase and anisoylated streptokinase plasminogen complex. Their action on haemostasis in human volunteers. Eur J Clin Pharmacol 1983; **24**:751–6.

56. Ferres H, Hibbs M, Smith RAG. Deacylation studies in vitro on anisoylated plasminogen streptokinase activator complex. Drugs 1987; **33**(suppl 3):80–2.

57. Nunn B, Esmail A, Fears R, Ferres H, Strandring R. Pharmacokinetic properties of anisoylated plasminogen streptokinase activator complex and other thrombolytic agents in animals and in humans. Drugs 1987; **33**(suppl 3):88–92.

58. Verstraete M. Thrombolytic treatment in acute myocardial infarction. Circulation 1990; **82**(suppl 3): II96–II109.

59. Hoffmann JJML, Bonnier JJRM, de Swart JBRM, Cutsers P, Vijgen M. Systemic effects of anisoylated plasminogen streptokinase activator complex and streptokinase therapy in acute myocardial infarction. Drugs 1987; **33**(suppl 3):242–6.

60. Jalihal S, Morris GK. Anti-streptokinase titers after intravenous streptokinase. Lancet 1990; **335**:184–5.

61. Collen D, Van de Werf F. Coronary thrombolysis with recombinant staphylokinase in patients with evolving myocardial infarction. Circulation 1993; **87**:1850–3.

62. Vanderschueren S, Barrios L, Kerdsinchai P et al. A randomized trial of recombinant staphylokinase versus alteplase for coronary artery patency in acute myocardial infarction. Circulation 1995; **92**:2044–9.

63. Armstrong P, Burton J, Palisaitis D et al. Collaborative angiographic patency trial of recombinant staphylokinase (CAPTORS). Am Heart J 2000; **139**:820–3.

64. Vanderschueren S, Collen D, Van de Werf F. A pilot study on bolus administration of recombinant staphylokinase for coronary artery thrombolysis. Thromb Haemost 1996; **76**:541–4.

65. Okada K, Lijnen HR, Moreau H, Vanderschueren S, Collen D. Procoagulant properties of intravenous staphylokinase versus tissue-type plasminogen activator. Thromb Haemost 1996; **76**:857–9.

2

General principles of fibrinolytic therapy in acute myocardial infarction

Robert G Wilcox

Introduction

Functional or mechanical impairment of endothelial integrity may lead stealthily to atherosclerotic plaque formation and acute episodes of vasospasm or localized intravascular thrombosis. In the coronary circulation the clinical consequences might be silent or symptomatic episodes of myocardial ischaemia, sometimes progressing over the years to an ischaemic cardiomyopathy or, in the presence of a critical flow-limiting thrombus, to more profound ischaemic events, such as unstable angina or myocardial necrosis if the occlusion is not relieved. The degree and consequences of myocardial necrosis (infarction) will depend on the vessel affected, the proximal site, extent and duration of the occlusion, the extent of other vessel disease and the quality of collateral coronary flow.

In patients with the clinical event of acute myocardial infarction, coronary artery thrombosis was proposed as the underlying pathological cause as early as 1912 by Herrick, but for decades thereafter it was regarded as an epiphenomenon or post-mortem artefact.[1] However, the demonstration of fresh occlusive thrombi at post-mortem and during acute angiography in preparation for coronary artery bypass surgery, eventually led to the acceptance that in the majority of patients with acute myocardial infarction the cause is occlusion by fresh platelet-rich thrombus in the vicinity of an eroded or fissured atherosclerotic plaque. Angiography showed the process may be dynamic, with spontaneous fibrinolysis and restoration of some coronary flow followed by reocclusion occurring over several hours, such that by 24 hours as many as 50% of presumed originally occluded vessels may be patent, albeit leaving irreversible ischaemic damage to myocardial cells.[2–5] Animal models of coronary occlusion revealed not only the time dependency of the histopathological extent of such ischaemic necrosis but also a peri-infarct zone of muscle potentially viable if reperfusion was re-established and the effects of reperfusion injury minimal.[6–8]

These experimental, pathological and clinical studies of the acute occlusive thrombotic cause of most instances of myocardial infarction, and the potential for damage limitation, coincided with a reawakened interest in the thrombolytic properties of streptokinase and other plasminogen activators, and a surge in understanding of the central role of platelets in acute arterial thrombus formation. Chemical dissolution of an occluding thrombus was soon shown to be feasible and relatively safe when administered by a peripheral vein rather than directly into the infarct-related coronary artery, and resulted in a significant reduction in both short- and long-term mortality. Effective proactive rather than reactive treatment of acute myocardial infarction had arrived.

Clinical opportunities

Acute total or subtotal occlusion of a coronary artery usually causes severe chest pain, sweating, haemodynamic instability and the threat of fatal dysrhythmias. The acute episode is most often accompanied by ECG changes of ST elevation over the area of threatened myocardium, or bundle branch block (usually left bundle). In subtotal or transient occlusion intermittent ST depression or T-wave inversion may occur. In this acute phase the patient is at high risk: some 30% die before admission to hospital and another 15% or more in hospital, such that by one month 40–50% of patients will have died. Of those who survive, a considerable proportion will be significantly disabled with reduced effort tolerance depending upon the extent of left ventricular (LV) damage and the quality of residual function. The risk of reinfarction in the next year varies considerably from ≤ 5% to ≥ 40% depending on age and other comorbidities, the extent of residual coronary artery disease and especially on the quantity and quality of residual LV function.[9]

These clinicopathological associations and the opportunity for damage limitation and improved prognosis, by restoration of coronary artery patency and myocardial perfusion, makes the assessment, protection (by defibrillator availability) and proactive treatment of a patient with acute myocardial infarction a medical emergency. The early reestablishment of infarct-related coronary artery patency is crucial. In one study, patients treated with thrombolytic therapy who had early and sustained restoration of patency had an in-hospital mortality of ≤ 5%, those with initial patency who reoccluded 10%, and those who failed to reopen at all a mortality of 17%.[10] In the clinical context of an evolving acute myocardial infarction, 'time costs muscle—and muscle buys time'.

Restoring vessel patency

There are currently two major options for restoring timely patency of an occluded coronary artery: immediate coronary angiography with a view to angioplasty and stent (or in some instances coronary artery bypass surgery), or chemical thrombolysis. For the majority of patients worldwide, chemical thrombolysis will be the only available option.

Thrombolytic drugs, of which the bacterially derived streptokinase is the archetype, work by enhancing the conversion of naturally occurring plasminogen within the circulation to the protease enzyme plasmin: they are not direct acting lytics of a thrombus; it is the generated plasmin that digests fibrinogen and fibrin, which, together with platelets, are the structural elements of occlusive thrombi (see Fig. 2.1). Rather than circulating plasminogen, that bound within an occluding thrombus is obviously a more attractive target for a thrombolytic drug, for this has the potential advantage of generating local clot-bound plasmin rather than a more systemic state of hyperplasminaemia and the associated increased risk of bleeding. Whereas streptokinase activates circulating plasminogen but has poor penetrance into thrombi, the next generation of bioengineered derivatives of naturally occurring (wild-type) tissue plasminogen activator (t-PA) have enhanced plasminogen activation in the presence of clot-bound thrombin with the potential for more concentrated local rather than systemic plasmin generation and activity. Such thrombolytics are termed 'clot-specific', although they do cause some systemic plasminogen conversion and do not differentiate between clots in different

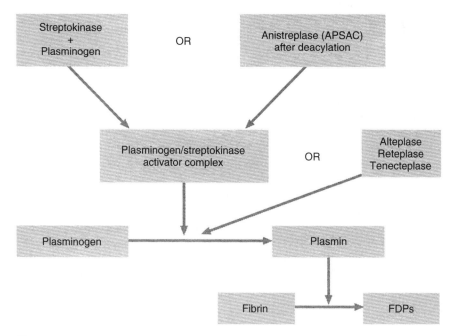

Figure 2.1

Thrombolytic activation of plasminogen.

vascular territories, a weakness which in part may be responsible for their most dangerous unwanted effect of intracerebral haemorrhage.

Of course, there are limitations to the effectiveness of thrombolytic therapy. For instance, a ruptured plaque within the infarct-related coronary artery may mechanically prevent prograde penetration of systemically formed plasmin or of an intravenously administered thrombolytic drug, or an extensive column of thrombus may spread not only distally from the site of the initial lesion but also proximally, perhaps impairing perfusion of branching collateral vessels. Such an extensive 'clot burden' may prove an unassailable obstacle to permeation of plasmin or thrombolytic drug. There is some possibility too that the constituents of an occlusive thrombus may vary with extent and time, making it less susceptible to digestion by plasmin. Hence the urgency to initiate thrombolytic treatment and the search for more effective alternative thrombolytic drugs and antithrombotic cotreatments.

Clinical trials of thrombolysis

General comments

Streptokinase was first used in acute myocardial infarction (AMI) in 1958; this was followed by a number of rather small inconclusive studies of varying dose schedules and reported bleeding risks and thus interest waned.[11] Following the pathological and acute angiographic reports described above and two small experiences of intracoronary streptokinase,[12,13] several large controlled phase III trials of streptokinase, streptokinase-plasminogen complex and recombinant tissue plasminogen activator were reported in the late 1980s.[14–17] All showed a reduction in early (28–35 day) mortality, irrespective of thrombolytic type, and emphasized the declining efficacy when thrombolysis was initiated late after symptom onset. In addition, the increased risk of bleeding, especially of intracerebral bleeds, and the allergic-hypotensive potential of streptokinase, were documented.

From these and other smaller controlled trials, a meta-analysis published in 1994 provided an overall assessment of the benefits and risks from thrombolytic therapy and indicated those patient features that might be associated with no benefit or even harm (Tables 2.1 and 2.2).[18] Overall, the survival benefit is modest, an extra 2–3 lives saved per 100 patients treated, albeit with an increased risk of total stroke of about 0.4%. These controlled trials were carried out at a time when image acquisition for stroke was not universal and the figures are probably underestimates. The benefit, however, is sustained over many years.[19]

Table 2.1 Overview of risk/benefit from thrombolysis in acute myocardial infarction.

	Control (%)	Fibrinolytic (%)
Mortality 35 days	11.5	9.6
Stroke 35 days[a]	0.8	1.2
Major bleeds[a]	0.4	1.1

[a] Majority in hospital. Adapted from the Fibrinolytic Therapy Trialists' Collaborative Group (1994).[18]

Table 2.2 Benefit from thrombolysis according to baseline demographic features.

Group	Control group death (%)	Benefit/1000 patients
Men	10.1	19
Women	16.0	18
Age		
< 55 years	4.6	11
55–64	8.9	18
65–74	16.1	27
> 75	25.3	10
Prior MI		
Yes	14.1	16
No	10.9	20
Diabetes		
Yes	17.3	37
No	10.2	15
ECG		
Bundle branch block	23.6	49
Anterior ST raised	16.9	37
Inferior ST raised	8.4	8
ST depression	13.8	−14
Other abnormal	5.8	6
Normal	2.3	−7

Adapted from the Fibrinolytic Therapy Trialists' Collaborative Group (1994).[18]

Adding aspirin

One substantial trial, ISIS-2, compared the efficacy of streptokinase, aspirin, both or neither in 17 187 patients.[15] The 35 day cardiovascular mortality according to treatment was 13.2% placebo, 10.4% streptokinase, 10.7% aspirin and 8.0% for combined aspirin plus streptokinase, a 5% absolute reduction in cardiovascular death (i.e. a saving of 5 lives per 100 patients treated). This pivotal trial led to aspirin, an antiplatelet drug by virtue of its inhibition of platelet cyclooxygenase, being recommended as initial cotreatment irrespective of which thrombolytic is used.

Improving treatment schedules

The next major step in thrombolytic therapy was the GUSTO-I trial, which compared streptokinase (with subcutaneous or intravenous heparin), and a newly described 90 min bolus-infusion 'accelerated' schedule of alteplase with intravenous heparin, and a combination arm of reduced dose streptokinase plus alteplase; all treatment groups included aspirin.[20,21] The 30 day overall mortality was a significant 1% (± 0.6%) lower with the alteplase schedule, thus giving the potential for a further small reduction in overall mortality. Unfortunately, the cost differential between streptokinase and alteplase prevented its widespread adoption as the preferred lytic.

The search for simpler treatment schedules: bolus thrombolytics

Tissue plasminogen activator (t-PA) is produced by vascular endothelium and is neutralized by plasminogen activator inhibitors. Alteplase (rt-PA) is the recombinant tissue plasminogen activator that is produced by recombinant DNA technology. Several derivatives of rt-PA have been synthesized and three of them (reteplase, lanoteplase and tenecteplase) compared with alteplase in phase III outcome studies. These derivatives vary minimally (tenecteplase) or substantially (reteplase) from the parent molecule, but the property they share in common and which has been exploited therapeutically is a longer half-life, permitting bolus rather than infusion administration (see Fig. 2.2). Tenecteplase, in addition, has some resistance to tissue plasminogen activator inhibitors. Both reteplase and lanoteplase lack the finger domain of the parent molecule and thus have lower affinities for fibrin than alteplase, whereas tenecteplase has more. Antigenicity has not been a problem with any of these new molecules.

The possibility of bolus administration of a thrombolytic drug increases the possibility of more rapid treatment after patient assessment in the receiving room, and the real opportunities for very early treatment in the community where most heart attacks occur.

Reteplase (r-PA)
The half-life of this bioengineered t-PA led to the investigation of double bolus intravenous injections separated by 30 min. After two coronary artery patency studies against 'original' 3 hour alteplase infusion and 'accelerated' 90 min alteplase (RAPIDS 1 and 2), a double bolus 10 MU schedule, separated by 30 min, was chosen for comparison with streptokinase in patients with AMI (INJECT study).[22] This was a pivotal trial in cardiovascular medicine, for it introduced the concept of equivalence of

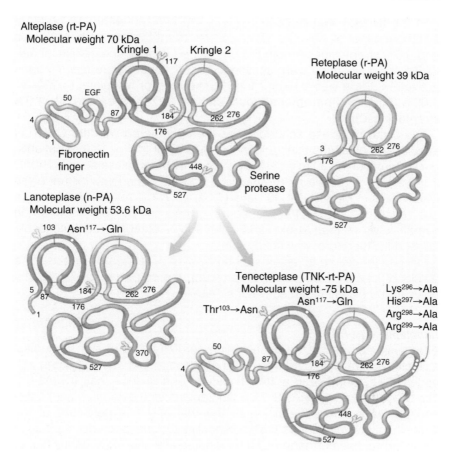

Figure 2.2

Structure of various thrombolytic agents. The structure–function relationships for the various domains are as follows: kringle 1, receptor binding (liver); kringle 2, fibrin binding (low affinity); fibronectin finger, fibrin binding (high affinity); epidermal growth factor, hepatic clearance; serine protease, catalytic activity and plasminogen activator inhibitor 1 binding; glycosylation sites, clearance via hepatic endothelial cells. Reproduced with permission from Llevadot et al (2001).[50]

efficacy between two drugs rather than an attempt to assert superiority. Equivalence has clinical as well as statistical boundaries and allows the testing of a new drug in a clinical situation where a placebo comparator would not be ethical. In the event that equivalence is proven, then in order to be preferred against a proven and long established comparator, the new drug must confer other advantages, such as ease of administration, lower cost or fewer unwanted effects.

In the INJECT trial of 6010 patients randomized within 12 hours of symptom onset of AMI, the 35 day mortality rates were 9.0% reteplase and 9.5% streptokinase, both the predefined clinical and statistical definition of equivalence were satisfied. As with other tissue plasminogen activators, there was a higher total stroke rate for reteplase (1.23% vs 1.00%) and comparable serious bleeds (0.7% reteplase vs 1.0% streptokinase).

The same reteplase schedule was then compared with the GUSTO-I accelerated alteplase schedule in the GUSTO-III trial of 15 059 patients, but because of the 90 min patency superiority of reteplase seen in RAPID 2 (59.9% vs 45.2%) a more ambitious survival superiority for reteplase was sought.[23] Mortality at 30 days (7.5% vs 7.2%, respectively) and at one year (11.2% vs 11.1%, respectively) were comparable, as were the overall rates of total stroke and other major bleeding complications. Superiority, therefore, was not proven.

Despite the failure to assert superiority over accelerated alteplase, the results of INJECT and GUSTO-III provided the cardiologist with the first bolus tissue plasminogen activator schedule.

Lanoteplase (n-PA)

After similar modest-sized dose-finding coronary artery patency studies, a single dose of 120 kU/kg dose of lanoteplase (n-PA) was compared with accelerated alteplase in a 15 078 patient equivalence trial, InTime-II.[24] The 30 day mortality rates (6.75% lanoteplase vs 6.61% alteplase) satisfied the equivalence definition of the trial and this persisted at the 6 month follow-up (8.7% vs 8.8%, respectively). Unexpectedly, the rate of intracerebral haemorrhage (ICH) for lanoteplase was significantly higher than for alteplase (1.12% vs 0.64%, $p = 0.004$), although this was the lowest ICH rate ever recorded for any alteplase trial with strict imaging acquisition and verification. There was also an increased incidence of minor bleeds with lanoteplase (19.7% vs 14.8%, $p < 0.0001$). Whatever the cause of the increased bleeding complications—the dose of lanoteplase, the heparin schedule, the age composition of the patient group or the lower fibrin specificity of lanoteplase—it was decided not to pursue the drug for therapeutic use. However, the lessons learnt from the follow-on smaller InTime-IIb lower heparin schedule study led to important changes for adjunctive heparin dosage and the recommendation for earlier assessment of the activated partial thromboplastin time by the American College of Cardiology/American Heart Association Guidelines Committee.

Tenecteplase (TNK-rt-PA)

In contrast with the modest-sized phase II dose-finding studies carried out with reteplase and lanoteplase, tenecteplase underwent extensive phase II patency and safety studies in the TIMI-IOB (837 patients) and ASSENT-1 (3325 patients) trials. An ICH rate of 0.62% was seen with the 40 mg dose combined with the now recommended lower heparin schedule.

The ASSENT-2 trial therefore compared a single bolus of tenecteplase 30–50 mg (depending on body weight) with accelerated alteplase in a 16 949 patient AMI trial.[25] Equivalent mortality rates were observed at 30 days (6.18% vs 6.15%) which persisted at 1 year. ICH rates, too, were comparable (0.93% tenecteplase vs 0.94% alteplase), although higher than hoped for from the phase II safety data.

Summary of bolus thrombolytic therapy

These three trials established the equivalent efficacy in terms of total mortality or the clinical composite of death plus non-fatal disabling stroke of gold standard accelerated alteplase and bolus therapy. They also ushered in new recommendations regarding heparin dosing and the timing of activated partial thromboplastin time (APTT) checks on its anticoagulant activity. Although lanoteplase has been abandoned, both reteplase and tenecteplase are now available as bolus therapies (double or single bolus alternatives) and are beginning to replace the more complex 90 min accelerated alteplase schedule. They are also being assessed (and promoted) as out-of-hospital thrombolytic treatments for patients in the very early throes of AMI where the greatest gains in mortality reduction (and possibly infarct abortion) are expected.

Vessel patency and microvascular perfusion

The goal of thrombolytic therapy is to achieve a patent infarct-related artery in the shortest possible time following symptom onset, with the lowest incidence of side-effects. In GUSTO-I a substantial angiographic substudy was carried out which confirmed the relationship between vessel patency and 30 day mortality (see Fig. 2.3); however, this was achieved in only 54% of patients with the most effective accelerated alteplase schedule.[26] Furthermore, early reocclusion occurs in 5–25% of treated patients depending on the thrombolytic and adjunctive thera-pies used.[26,27] Thus, the establishment and maintenance of early patency became the 'holy grail' of thrombolytic therapy, indeed of any reperfusion therapy. Despite the encouraging phase II superior early patency data obtained with the third-generation bolus thrombolytics (reteplase, lanoteplase and tenecteplase) described earlier, none have reduced mortality beyond that already achieved with accelerated alteplase. However, their ease of administration will ensure a role in the very early pre-hospital treatment area, a therapeutic opportunity largely

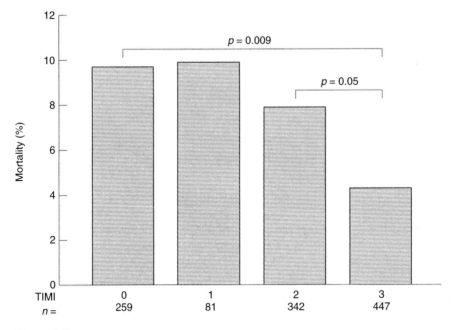

Figure 2.3

The 90 min TIMI patency grade and 30 day mortality following thrombolysis for acute myocardial infarction. From the GUSTO Angiographic Investigators (1993).[26]

ignored despite some optimistic earlier studies and local pockets of enthusiasm.[28]

Part of the explanation for this discrepancy came from studies in which myocardial perfusion was assessed in addition to epicardial vessel patency.[29,30] Between 25% and 50% of patients may have suboptimal perfusion despite optimal patency, the so-called 'no reflow phenomenon'.[31] This has complex causes that include microvascular emboli, microvascular oedema and the release of leucocyte cytokines.[32] In the search for speedier, more sustained vessel patency and improved microvascular perfusion, attention therefore shifted towards more powerful concomitant antithrombin and antiplatelet therapies. Thus, large phase II/III trials with enoxaparin, a low molecular weight heparin (ASSENT-3), abciximab, a platelet glycoprotein (GP) IIb/IIIa receptor blocker (ASSENT-3, GUSTO-V), and hirudin, a direct-acting antithrombin (HERO-2) have all been conducted and will be described in detail in subsequent chapters. Suffice here to say that none reduced the incidence of total mortality beyond that of established comparator thrombolytic schedules, nor of haemorrhagic stroke, but there were encouraging reductions of recurrent in-hospital ischaemic events, the clinical significance of which will only emerge with longer follow-up data.

Problems with thrombolytics

Stroke

The excess stroke risk which accompanies thrombolytic use is due to ICH, usually occurring within the first 24 hours and resulting in death in about 60% of affected patients, thereby contributing significantly to the overall mortality in treated patients and limiting the full potential of thrombolytic therapy. Hopes that haemorrhagic stroke risk would be reduced by the use of 'clot-specific' tissue plasminogen activator derivatives were dashed by several subsequent 'head-to-head' comparator trials described above. In general, haemorrhagic stroke risk after streptokinase is ≤ 0.5% and after a tissue plasminogen activator is 0.5–1.0%. The complicity of concomitant antithrombotic therapy with heparin in these events is an ongoing debate.[33] From the demographic and outcome data available from the thrombolytic trials, Simoons and colleagues published a model from which it may be possible to predict the likely risk of ICH.[34] Although this has not been tested prospectively, some clinicians refer to it when choosing between streptokinase and tissue plasminogen activators, or avoiding thrombolysis altogether, for instance, in a low-weight elderly lady with a 'small' inferior infarction.

Bleeding

Giving a thrombolytic drug, an antiplatelet and an antithrombin obviously increases the bleeding risk (Table 2.1), especially if the APTT is allowed to drift too high. Bleeds may occur spontaneously anywhere, but are more likely in the presence of covert bleeding areas (bowel, bladder) and especially at the sites of vascular puncture. The majority, however, are minor ecchymoses: the most serious, endangering life or neurological function, are intracranial bleeds, as described earlier.

Anaphylaxis

This occurs rarely in patients treated with a tissue plasminogen activator, but in ≤ 2% of patients given streptokinase. It is usually mild but can be life threatening in the event of a severe acute autoimmune-type response. Hypotension may occur in ≤ 10% of streptokinase-treated patients and can usually be treated with temporary cessation of the infusion (or switch to a tissue plasminogen activator if available), fluid replacement and atropine if associated with a bradycardia. Antibodies to streptokinase may last many years and theoretically could negate the benefit of further exposure or provoke an anaphylactic reaction.[35] In ideal circumstances, streptokinase should be a 'once-in-a-lifetime' drug.[36]

Failed thrombolysis and 'rescue'

It may be difficult to assert whether or not thrombolysis has been successful. If the patient remains in pain and the ECG shows persistent ST-segment elevation, then either patency or reperfusion has not been achieved. Schröder and colleagues promoted the principle of ST-segment elevation resolution (i.e. return to the isoelectric line, arbitrarily divided into no resolution, ≤ 30% resolution and ≥ 70% resolution).[37] This procedure was tested prospectively and compared with angiographic evidence of both patency (and later with perfusion too) and subsequently mortality (see Fig. 2.4).[31,38] Despite the excellent correlation, there remains no convincing trial evidence about which strategy to adopt—treat symptomatically with analgesia, antiischaemic and anticoagulant therapy, or a repeat trial of thrombolysis, or proceed to coronary angiography with a view to intervention. Limited controlled and uncontrolled data suggest that the latter policy is excellent if the intervention is successful, but disastrous if it's not![39] Fortunately, there are other trials in progress randomizing patients to one of these three alternatives based on the degree of ST-segment elevation resolution as proposed by Schröder.

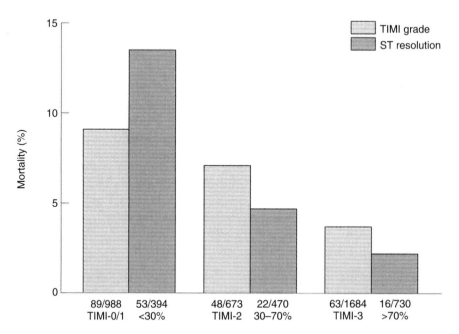

Figure 2.4

'Open artery' versus 'relief of ischaemia'. TIMI perfusion grades 0, 1, 2, 3 is assessment of coronary patency, and < 30%, 30–70%, > 70% assessment of ST-segment resolution. From Schröder et al (1995).[38]

After thrombolysis, then what?

All patients recovering from an acute myocardial infarction should be actively considered for prophylactic treatment with a number of proven therapies—aspirin, an angiotensin-converting enzyme (ACE) inhibitor, beta blocker, a statin and, in selected patients, spironolactone or similar aldosterone antagonist. The usefulness of long-term antiinflammatory therapy is not yet proven. The role of routine early exercise testing in the asymptomatic patient remains controversial, but there is some evidence provided a coronary intervention can be offered.[40,41]

Patient selection for thrombolytic therapy

The Fibrinolytic Therapy Trialists' (FTT) overview suggested that of those patients deemed initially eligible for thrombolysis (i.e. not considered to have a significant bleeding risk), the groups not likely to benefit were those whose initial electrocardiogram was either normal, equivocal, or showed ECG ST-segment depression rather than elevation (Tables 2.1 and 2.2). Even in the elderly, some overall benefit was retained, although in the context of general use rather than in the context of a clinical trial setting, this assertion has been challenged.[42]

The maximum potential from a thrombolytic strategy is likely only to be realized if treatment can be started as soon as possible after symptom onset (see Fig. 2.5).[43] This would necessitate a significant reduction in the patient delay to calling for medical assistance, a rapid medical response, and the initiation of treatment out-of-hospital, either by paramedic personnel or attending primary care physicians. The availability now of bolus rather than intravenous infusion thrombolytic schedules makes pre-hospital thrombolysis an urgent priority for widespread implementation.

In general, in the absence of an experienced immediately available primary angioplasty service, thrombolysis should be considered for every patient presenting within 12 hours of onset of chest pain considered to be due to myocardial ischaemia and whose ECG shows either ST elevation or bundle branch block (thought to be new, but often difficult to be certain in practice). Beyond 12 hours there may be little myocardium left to 'salvage', but in the presence of continuing pain and ST elevation and the uncertainty of the timing of infarction, offering thrombolytic treatment would seem reasonable.

It is not reasonable, however, to withhold thrombolysis in a patient with proliferative diabetic retinopathy or after cardiopulmonary resuscitation, but in the presence of hypotension an alternative to streptokinase is to be preferred lest further blood pressure lowering occurs. In view of the uncertain consequences of streptokinase antibodies in a previously

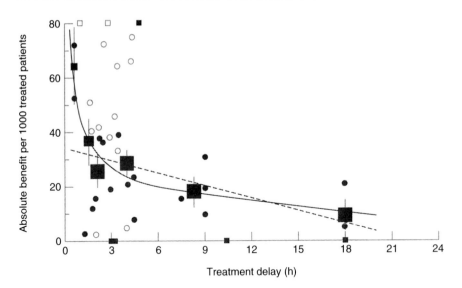

Figure 2.5

Relationship between treatment delay and absolute benefit per 1000 treated patients.
Symbols represent the results of individual trials entered in the analysis. Reproduced with
permission from the Lancet (1996).[43]

treated patient, it is probably prudent to avoid re-exposure at all if alternative drugs are available. Even if re-administered within 48 hours before significant antibodies appear its therapeutic use may be reduced by virtue of low plasma plasminogen which was 'consumed' by the earlier dose.

Clinical guidelines and treatment schedules

For common clinical guidelines and contraindications see Table 2.3, but also review the information inserts for a particular product.[44] Of the contraindications listed some may be of lesser risk than others and for some clear evidence lacking, so clinical judgement will often be needed. A history of hypertension but with preliminary good control and 'normal' value on admission or a previously normotensive patient with elevated levels on admission, whether or not reduced by medical therapy, remain difficult judgement issues. In the absence of easily available alternative therapy with percutaneous transluminal coronary angioplasty (PTCA), then streptokinase (if previously not given) might be the lytic of choice, but even its information insert gives ambiguous advice. If clinical judgement suggests that the intracerebral bleeding risk is higher than the expected benefit, then the lytic should be withheld.

Current fibrinolytic schedules are given in Table 2.4; all include cotreatment with oral aspirin.[44] Adjunctive treatment with heparin has never been proven to reduce mortality irrespective of fibrinolytic drug used. It is

Table 2.3 Thrombolysis in acute myocardial infarction: indications and contraindications.

Indications
Clinical presentation consistent with myocardial infarction within the previous 12 h and at least one of:
- 1 mm ST elevation in two or more contiguous limb leads
- 2 mm ST elevation in two or more contiguous limb leads
- New (presumed or known) left bundle branch block
- Consider in patients presenting 12–24 h if chest pain and ST elevation are persisting

Absolute contraindications[a]
- Haemorrhage stroke or stroke of unknown origin at any time
- Ischaemic stroke in preceding 6 months
- Central nervous system damage or neoplasms
- Recent major trauma/surgery/head injury within preceding 3 weeks
- Gastrointestinal bleeding within the last month
- Known bleeding disorder
- Aortic dissection

Relative contraindications[a]
- Transient ischaemic attack in preceding 6 months
- Oral anticoagulant therapy
- Pregnancy or within 1 week post-partum
- Non-compressible vascular punctures
- Traumatic resuscitation
- Refractory hypertension (systolic blood pressure > 180 mmHg)
- Advanced liver disease
- Infective endocarditis
- Active peptic ulcer

[a] From the Task Force on the Management of Acute Myocardial Infarction of the European Society of Cardiology (2003).[44]

Table 2.4 Fibrinolytic regimens for acute myocardial infarction.

Fibrinolytic	Initial treatment	Antithrombin	Contraindications
Streptokinase	1.5 million units in 100 ml 5% dextrose or 0.9% saline over 30–60 min	None or i.v. heparin for 24–48 h	Prior streptokinase or anistreplase
Alteplase	15 mg i.v. bolus 0.75 mg kg^{-1} over 30 min i.v. 0.5 mg kg^{-1} over 60 min i.v. Total dose ≤ 100 mg	i.v. heparin for 24–48 h	
Reteplase	10 U + 10 U i.v. bolus given 30 min apart	i.v. heparin for 24–48 h	
Tenecteplase	single i.v. bolus of 30 mg if < 60 kg 35 mg if 60 kg to < 70 kg 40 mg if 70 kg to < 80 kg 45 mg if 80 kg to < 90 kg 50 mg if ≥ 90 kg	i.v. heparin for 24–48 h	

From the Task Force on the Management of Acute Myocardial Infarction of the European Society of Cardiology (2003).[44]

recommended especially in conjunction with a tissue plasminogen activator (alteplase, reteplase, tenecteplase) purely on the basis of phase II coronary artery patency trials. The optimal dose, duration and anticoagulant intensity are not known, but recent advice would be to monitor APTT early, to keep within 55–70 seconds and to employ weight adjustment normograms.[33] These regimens may change according to local interpretation of trials incorporating low-dose heparin, direct-acting antithrombins, or platelet glycoprotein (GP) IIb/IIIa inhibitors.

Concluding comments

Thrombolytic therapy with concomitant aspirin (and possibly heparin) has reduced the risk of death in eligible patients by about 40%. There are problems concerning the time delay between symptom onset and treatment prescription which can only be resolved by out-of-hospital therapy. The cheapest drug, streptokinase, does have antigenic potential and is not ideally suitable for pre-hospital treatment as an infusion, but the newer bolus lytics are (reteplase and tenecteplase). Whereas aspirin cotreatment seems essential, other adjunctive therapies remain to be proven and will be discussed in the following chapters. The issue of risk, especially from intracranial haemorrhage, undoubtedly has a negative impact on prescribing behaviour in some countries more than others, but what remains inexplicable is the underuse of lytics in apparently lytic-eligible patients.[45,46] Whereas 50% or more of patients with acute myocardial infarction appear eligible for thrombolysis, up to a quarter of them do not receive it or any other reperfusion therapy and have a higher mortality.[47] Finally, a significant proportion of patients are considered ineligible for thrombolysis and without the option of coronary angioplasty or timely coronary artery bypass surgery these patients have long been known to have a mortality several fold higher than thrombolysed patients.[48,49] To date there have been few attempts to test alternative strategies in this heterogeneous very high-risk group of patients.

References

1. Herrick JB. Clinical features of sudden obstruction of the coronary arteries. JAMA 1912; **59**:2015–20.

2. Davies MJ, Woolf N, Robertson NB. Pathology of acute myocardial infarction with particular reference to occlusive coronary thrombi. Br Heart J 1976; **38**:659–64.

3. Bertrand ME, Lefebure JM, Laine CL. Coronary angiography in acute transmural myocardial infarction. Am Heart J 1979; **97**:61–9.

4. DeWood MA, Spores J, Notske R et al. Prevalence of total coronary occlusion during the early hours of

transmural myocardial infarction. N Engl J Med 1980; **303**:897–902.

5. Falk E. Plaque rupture with severe pre-existing stenosis precipitating coronary thrombosis. Characteristics of coronary atherosclerotic plaques underlying fatal occlusive thrombi. Br Heart J 1983; **50**:127–34.

6. Tennant R, Wiggers CJ. The effects of coronary occlusion on myocardial contraction. Am J Physiol 1935; **112**:351–61.

7. Reimer KA, Lowe JE, Rasmussen MM, Jennings RB. The wavefront phenomenon of ischaemic cell death: 1. Myocardial infarct size vs duration of coronary occlusion in dogs. Circulation 1977; **56**: 786–94.

8. Yellon DM, Hearse DJ, Crome R, Wyse RKH. Temporal and spatial characteristics of evolving cell injury during regional myocardial ischaemia in the dog: the "borderline zone" controversy. J Am Coll Cardiol 1983; **2**:661–70.

9. White HD, Norris RM, Brown MA et al. Effects of intravenous streptokinase on left ventricular function and early survival after acute myocardial infarction. N Engl J Med 1987; **317**:850–5.

10. Ohman EM, Califf RM, Topol EJ et al. Consequences of reocclusion after successful reperfusion therapy in acute myocardial infarction. TAMI Study Group. Circulation 1990; **82**:781–91.

11. Fletcher AP, Alkjaersig N, Smyrniotis FE et al. Treatment of patients suffering from early myocardial infarction with massive and prolonged streptokinase therapy. Trans Assoc Am Phys 1958; **71**:287–96.

12. Chazov EI, Matveeva LS, Mazaev AV, Sargin KE, Sadovskaia GV, Ruda MI. Acute myocardial infarction: intracoronary administration of fibrinolysis in acute myocardial infarction. Ter Arkh 1976; **48**:8–19.

13. Rentrop KP, Blanke H, Karsch KR et al. Acute myocardial infarction: intracoronary applications of nitroglycerin and streptokinase. Clin Cardiol 1979; **2**:354–63.

14. Gruppo Italiano per lo Studio della Streptochinasi nell'Infarto Miocardico. Effectiveness of intravenous thrombolytic treatment in acute myocardial infarction. Lancet 1986; **1**:397–402.

15. ISIS-2 (Second International Study of Infarct Survival) Collaborative Group. Randomised trial of intravenous streptokinase, oral aspirin, both or neither among 17,187 cases of suspected acute myocardial infarction: ISIS-2. Lancet 1988; **ii**:349–60.

16. AIMS Trial Study Group. Effect of intravenous APSAC on mortality after acute myocardial infarction: preliminary report of a placebo controlled clinical trial. Lancet 1988; **31**:545–9.

17. Wilcox RG, Von der Lippe G, Olsson CG, Jensen G, Skene AM, Hampton JR. Trial of tissue plasminogen activator for mortality reduction in acute myocardial infarction. Anglo-Scandinavian Study of Early Thrombolysis (ASSET). Lancet 1988; **2**:525–30.

18. Fibrinolytic Therapy Trialists' (FTT) Collaborative Group. Indications for fibrinolytic therapy in suspected acute myocardial infarction: collaborative overview of early mortality and major morbidity results from all randomised trials of more than 1000 patients. Lancet 1994; **343**:311–22.

19. Franzosi MG, Santoro E, De Vita C et al. Ten year follow up of the first megatrial testing thromboloytic therapy in patients with acute myocardial infarction. Results of the Gruppo Italiano per lo Studio della Sopravvivenza

nell'Infarcto-1 Study. Circulation 1998; **98**:2659–65.

20. Neuhaus KL, Von Essen R, Tebbe U et al. Improved thrombolysis in acute myocardial infarction with front-loaded administration of alteplase: results of the rt-PA-APSAC patency study (TAPS). J Am Coll Cardiol 1992; **19**:885–91.

21. GUSTO investigators. An international randomised trial comparing four thrombolytic strategies for acute myocardial infarction. N Engl J Med 1993; **329**:673–82.

22. INJECT Study Group. International Joint Efficacy Comparison of Thrombolytics. Randomised, double-blind comparison of Reteplase double-bolus administration with streptokinase in acute myocardial infarction (INJECT): a trial to investigate equivalence. Lancet 1995; **346**:329–36.

23. GUSTO-III: Global Use of Strategies to Open Occluded Coronary Arteries investigators. A comparison of Reteplase with Alteplase for acute myocardial infarction. N Engl J Med 1997; **337**:1118–23.

24. InTime-II Investigators. Intravenous n-PA for the treatment of infarcting myocardium early. InTime-II, a double-blind comparison of single-bolus Lanoteplase vs accelerated Alteplase for the treatment of patients with acute myocardial infarction. Eur Heart J 2000; **21**:2005–13.

25. Assessment of the Safety and Efficacy of a New Thrombolytic Investigators. Single bolus Tenecteplase compared with front-loaded Alteplase in acute myocardial infarction: the ASSENT-2 double-blind randomised trial. Lancet 1999; **354**:716–22.

26. GUSTO Angiographic investigators. The effects of tissue plasminogen activator, streptokinase, or both on coronary artery patency, ventricular function and survival after acute myocardial infarction. N Engl J Med 1993; **329**:1615–22.

27. Meijer A, Verheught FW, Werter CJ, Lie KI, Van der Pol JM, Van Eenige MJ. Aspirin versus coumadin in the prevention of reocclusion and recurrent ischaemia after successful thrombolysis: a prospective placebo-controlled angiographic study. Results of the APRICOT Study. Circulation 1993; **87**:1524–30.

28. Rawles J. Halving of mortality at 1 year by domiciliary thrombolysis in the Grampian Region Early Anistreplase Trial (GREAT). J Am Coll Cardiol 1994; **23**:1–5.

29. Ito M, Tomooka T, Sakai N et al. A lack of myocardial perfusion immediately after successful thrombolysis: a predictor of poor recovery of left ventricular function in anterior myocardial infarction. Circulation 1992; **85**: 1699–705.

30. Maes A, Van der Werf F, Nuyts J et al. Impaired myocardial tissue perfusion early after successful thrombolysis. Impact on myocardial flow, metabolism and function at late follow up. Circulation 1995; **92**:2072–8.

31. Gibson CM, Cannon CP, Murphy SA et al. Relationship of TIMI Myocardial Perfusion Grade to mortality after administration of thrombolytic drugs. Circulation 2000; **101**:125–30.

32. Verma S, Fedak P, Weisel R et al. Fundamentals of reperfusion injury for the clinical cardiologist. Circulation 2002; **105**:2332–6.

33. Giugliano RP, McCabe CH, Antman EM et al. The Thrombolysis in Myocardial Infarction

(TIMI) Investigators. Lower dose heparin with fibrinolysis is associated with lower rates of intracranial haemorrhage. Am Heart J 2001; **141**:742–50.

34. Simoons ML, Maggioni AP, Knatterud G et al. Individual risk assessment for intracranial haemorrhage during thrombolytic therapy. Lancet 1993; **342**: 1523–8.

35. Squire IB, Lawley W, Fletcher S et al. Humoral and cellular responses up to 7.5 years after administration of streptokinase for acute myocardial infarction. Eur Heart J 1999; **20**:1245–52.

36. Jennings K. Antibodies to streptokinase. BMJ 1996; **312**:393–4.

37. Schröder R, Dissman R, Brüggermann T, Wegscheider K, Linderer T, Tebbe U. Extent of early ST segment elevation resolution: a simple but strong predictor of outcome in patients with acute myocardial infarction. J Am Coll Cardiol 1994; **24**:384–91.

38. Schröder R, Wegscheider K, Schröder K, Dissmann R, Meyer-Sabellek W for the INJECT Trial Group. Extent of early ST segment elevation resolution: a strong predictor of outcome in patients with acute myocardial infarction and a sensitive measure to compare thrombolytic regimes. J Am Coll Cardiol 1995; **26**:1657–64.

39. Barbash GI, Birnbaum Y, Bogaerts K et al. Treatment of reinfarction after thrombolytic therapy for acute myocardial infarction: an analysis of outcome and treatment choices in the global utilisation of streptokinase and tissue plasminogen activator for occluded coronary arteries (GUSTO-I) and assessment of the safety of a new thrombolytic (ASSENT-2) studies. Circulation 2001; **103**:954–60.

40. Villella A, Maggioni AP, Villella M et al on behalf of the GISSI-2 Investigators. Prognostic significance of maximal exercise testing after myocardial infarction treated with thrombolytic agents: the GISSI-2 data-base. Lancet 1995; **346**:523–9.

41. Madsen JK, Grande P, Saunamaki K et al. Danish Multicenter Randomised Study of Invasive Versus Conservative Treatment in Patients with Inducible Ischemia After Thrombolysis in Acute Myocardial Infarction (DANAMI). Circulation 1997; **96**:748–55.

42. Thiemann DR, Coresh J, Schulman P et al. Lack of benefit of intravenous thrombolysis in patients with myocardial infarction who are older than 75 years. Circulation 2000; **101**:2239–46.

43. Boersma E, Maas AC, Deckers JW, Simoons ML. Early thrombolytic treatment in acute myocardial infarction: reappraisal of the golden hour. Lancet 1996; **348**:771–5.

44. Task Force on the Management of Acute Myocardial Infarction of the European Society of Cardiology. Management of acute myocardial infarction in patients presenting with ST-segment elevation. Eur Heart J 2003; **24**:28–66.

45. Hillegass WB, Jollis GJ, Granger CB, Ohman EM, Califf RM, Mark DB. Intracranial hemorrhage risk and new thrombolytic therapies in acute myocardial infarction. Am J Cardiol 1994; **73**:444–9.

46. Weaver WD. The role of thrombolytic drugs in the management of myocardial infarction. Comparative clinical trials. Eur Heart J 1996; **17**(suppl F):9–15.

47. Rogers WJ, Canto JG, Lambrew CT et al for the Investigators in the National Registry of Myocardial Infarction 1, 2 and 3.

Temporal trends in the treatment of over 1.5 million patients with myocardial infarction in the US from 1990 through 1999. J Am Coll Cardiol 2000; **36**:2056–63.

48. Grines CL, DeMaria AN. Optimal utilisation of thrombolytic therapy for acute myocardial infarction: concepts and controversies. J Am Coll Cardiol 1990; **16**: 223–31.

49. Norris RM on behalf of the UK Heart Attack Study Investigators. Sudden cardiac death and acute myocardial infarction in three British Health Districts: the UK Heart Attack Study. London: British Heart Foundation, 1999.

50. Llevadot J, Giugliano RP, Autman EM. Bolus fibrinolytic therapy in acute myocardial infarction. JAMA 2001; **286**:442–9.

3
Antiplatelet therapy

Gianluca Gonzi, Silvia Buratti and Diego Ardissino

Introduction

Antiplatelet therapy is important in the treatment of acute coronary syndromes because it significantly reduces the incidence of major coronary events and ischaemic complications. The therapeutic approach to coronary diseases concentrates on the pathophysiological mechanisms underlying intracoronary thrombosis, a process in which platelets play a pivotal role, and which can be efficaciously controlled and prevented by antiplatelet therapy. Coronary thrombosis may occur unexpectedly at any stage in the evolution of atherosclerotic disease: it may represent the initial phase of plaque growth and repair (and thus cause the onset or worsening of angina), or lead to a partial or complete occlusion of the coronary lumen that is clinically manifested as an acute coronary syndrome.

The treatment of ischaemic heart disease involves the use of anti-ischaemic and antithrombotic drugs, mainly antiplatelet and anticoagulant agents. Aspirin and ticlopidine are cornerstones in the treatment of acute coronary syndromes. Particular attention has recently been given to the development of new antiplatelet agents, such as the glycoprotein (GP) IIb/IIIa inhibitors and clopidogrel, whose widespread use has demonstrated their efficacy in improving the outcome of patients with acute coronary syndromes and reducing the ischaemic complications associated with percutaneous revascularization procedures.

Pathogenesis

The initial mechanism in the pathogenesis of acute coronary syndromes, and which is responsible for starting the thrombotic process, is fissuring and/or rupture of the atheromatous plaque, and the subsequent exposure of subendothelial collagen and the lipidic core.[1,2] These components are potent stimulants of platelet activation and highly thrombogenic, a process that leads to a reduction in coronary flow.[3]

The interaction of platelets with the vessel wall, together with their contribution to the formation of atheromatous plaque and the thrombotic process, play a major role in the pathogenesis of coronary disease. The integrity of the vascular endothelium is fundamental in preventing the onset and progression of vascular thrombosis, which is otherwise amplified by the endothelial wall damage caused by atheromatous plaque rupture, the entry of thrombogenic substances into the blood flow and the interaction of platelets with coagulation factors.

Endothelial damage leads to the immediate deposit of platelets on the damaged wall by means of a mechanism of adhesion to the various components of the subendothelial connective matrix, including fibrin, collagen and laminin.[4] This process of platelet adhesion is initially mediated by von Willebrand's factor (vWF), a glycosylated multimeric protein that is synthesized by the endothelium and secreted into the subendothelium where it binds to collagen. Other plasma factors, such as fibronectin, fibrinogen and thrombospondin, are also directly involved in platelet adhesion. This adhesion and its recognition by platelets essentially depends on specific membrane platelet glycoproteins. Glycoprotein Ib platelet receptors bind to vWF, the main glycoprotein involved in the initial contact of platelets with the vessel wall. Platelet adhesion is also influenced by haemodynamic flow conditions: the presence of high wall shear stress potentiates platelet adhesion and subsequent activation.[5]

Platelet activation occurs after adhesion and may be induced by a large number of biochemical stimuli, the most powerful of which include the presence of thrombin, and platelet adhesion to collagen and the other components of the subendothelial matrix.

After platelets have adhered to the subendothelial matrix and thus become activated, they undergo a conformational modification that leads to the exposure of previously unexpressed GP IIb/IIIa platelet receptors, and the simultaneous release of the various substances contained in the platelet granules—serotonin, thromboxane A2, adenosine 5'-diphosphate (ADP), epinephrine (adrenaline)—which are capable of activating additional platelets.

The common final pathway leading to the formation of a platelet thrombus is platelet aggregation. Further platelet recruitment depends on the exposure of the GP IIb/IIIa receptor, which is only possible after the conformational modifications undergone by previously activated platelets. This receptor mainly binds to fibrinogen, a key component of the aggregation process insofar as it determines the formation of molecular bridges between the GP IIb/IIIa receptors of adjacent platelets, binding them together in a step that precedes thrombus formation and which progressively extends as further platelets are recruited and activated (Fig. 3.1). Unless controlled and regulated by compensatory mechanisms, the process may lead to the occlusion of the coronary lumen. This event is prevented by the antiaggregant substances—prostacyclin, endothelial-derived relaxing factor (EDRF), nitric oxide (NO) and ADPase—secreted by neighbouring undamaged endothelial cells.[6]

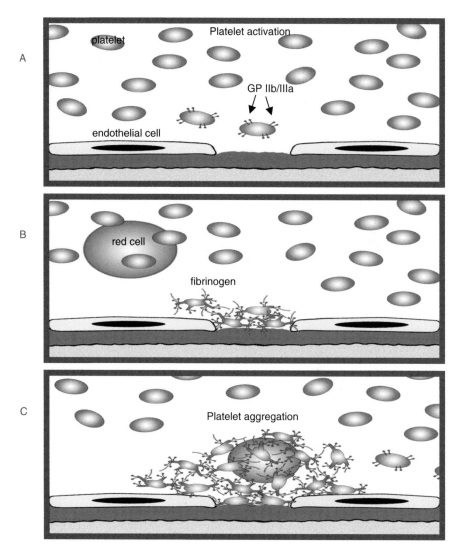

Figure 3.1

Platelet activation (A) causes changes in the shape of platelets and conformational changes in GP IIb/IIIa receptors, transforming the receptors from a ligand-unreceptive to a ligand-receptive state. GP IIb/IIIa-activated receptors bind fibrinogen molecules, which form bridges between adjacent platelets (B) and facilitate platelet aggregation (C).

However, the platelet thrombus is relatively unstable and only causes an initial obstruction of coronary flow. It is the endothelial damage that activates the coagulation cascade, which starts when tissue factor comes into contact with various circulating factors and ends with the formation of the fibrin that stabilizes the primary platelet thrombus. After its self-amplification, tissue factor forms an additional complex with factor X of the coagulation cascade on the surface of the activated platelets, whose membranes contain phospholipids capable of sustaining and potentiating the cascade by means of an intrinsic pathway. After its activation, factor X reassembles with complex V, but this is not capable of converting pro-thrombin into thrombin. The mechanism activating factor V (and therefore leading to the formation of thrombin) is not fully understood, but it is believed that a feedback mechanism allows moderate prothrombin levels to activate factor V which, by complexing with factor Xa, is capable of generating thrombin.[7] All of these reactions occur on the surfaces of activated platelets. Thrombin-mediated platelet activation can also be considered a positive feedback mechanism that increases thrombin levels and leads to thrombus formation. Thrombin plays a key role in the recruitment of additional platelets because it is *per se* the most potent physiological platelet activator.[8]

Thrombin subsequently catalyses the conversion of fibrinogen to fibrin, a filamentous protein that can bind to other monomers in order to form a stratified reticulum capable of trapping blood cells: a fibrin thrombus.

Acute phase of myocardial infarction

Aspirin

Aspirin inhibits prostaglandin G/H synthase (PGHS), the cyclooxygenase enzyme that catalyses the first step of the conversion of arachidonic acid to thromboxane A2, one of the more than 90 substances inducing platelet aggregation. Two isozymes of PGHS are known: $PGHS_1$ is expressed in virtually all human body cells, whereas $PGHS_2$ is undetectable in most mammalian tissues, but its expression can be induced in monocytes, endothelial cells and other specialized cells in response to various inflam-matory and mitogen mediators. The inhibition of PGHS by aspirin is permanent in platelets, because they are unable to generate new cyclooxygenase (Fig. 3.2).

The mechanism of action of aspirin is related to conformational changes in the structure of the active site of PGHS. The carboxylic moiety of salicylic acid acetylates the hydroxyl group of a serine residue at posi-tion 529 in the polypeptide chain of human platelet PGHS; when this happens, the acetyl group protrudes into the cyclooxygenase channel at a critical site for arachidonic acid interaction with the tyrosine residue responsible for initiating catalysis.

Orally ingested aspirin is rapidly absorbed by the stomach and the upper small intestine primarily by means of the passive diffusion of non-dissociated lipid-soluble aspirin, and partially as salicylate. The absorbed ester is rapidly hydrolysed to salicylate in plasma, the liver, lungs and erythrocytes. Salicylate is further metabolized mainly to salicyluric acid

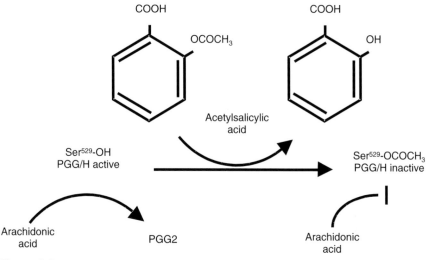

COOH

OCOCH₃

Acetylsalicylic
acid

COOH

OH

Ser⁵²⁹-OH
PGG/H active

Ser⁵²⁹-OCOCH₃
PGG/H inactive

Arachidonic
acid

PGG2

Arachidonic
acid

Figure 3.2

The main source of the eicosanoids (prostaglandins, thromboxanes and leukotrienes) is arachidonic acid, which is metabolized by one of two fatty acid cyclooxygenases and various lipoxygenases. Cyclooxygenase has two actions: the first is due to endoperoxide synthase that oxygenates arachidonate and is followed by cyclization to give the cyclic endoperoxide PGG2; the second is a peroxidase action that converts PGG2 to another cyclic endoperoxide, PGH2. The main action of acetylsalicylic acid is the inhibition of cyclooxygenase: it irreversibly inactivates the enzyme, acetylates serine⁵²⁹ at the apex of the COX-1 long hydrophobic channel (the main cyclooxygenase site) and thereby excludes arachidonic acid from the channel.

and partly to ester or acyl glucuronide; a small fraction is oxidized to gentisic acid and other metabolites without pharmacological effects. Salicylates are excreted mainly by the kidneys. The plasma half-life of aspirin is approximately 15 min, whereas that of salicylate is dose-dependent and ranges from 2 to 12 hours.

Aspirin is generally considered to be a weak platelet antagonist, but its therapeutic results are better than those of far more potent antiplatelet agents with potentially greater clinical effectiveness. ISIS-2 conclusively showed that the administration of aspirin 160 mg/day alone decreases 35 day mortality and reinfarction by 23% in acute myocardial infarction (AMI) patients and, when combined with streptokinase, decreases short-term mortality and reinfarction by 42%.[9] Since then, aspirin has become the gold standard of care for patients with myocardial infarction.

In the acute phase of myocardial infarction (MI) treated with thrombolytic agents, aspirin has been compared with oral anticoagulants in two trials: the Antithrombotics in the Prevention of Reocclusion In Coronary Thrombolysis (APRICOT), and the Aspirin/Anticoagulants Following Thrombolysis with Eminase in Recurrent Infarction (AFTER) studies.

The end-point of the APRICOT study was the 3 month reocclusion rate of a patent infarct-related artery demonstrated at angiography up to 48 hours after thrombolytic MI therapy. Reocclusion occurred in about 30% of the patients regardless of the use of antithrombotics. There was a reduced rate of reinfarction and revascularization in the aspirin group in comparison with the coumadin or placebo groups.[10] In the AFTER study, the 30 day and 3 month rates of cardiac death and recurrent MI were similar in the anticoagulant and aspirin groups (respectively, 11% and 13.2% vs 11.2% and 12.1%). The trial was stopped early because of its declining enrolment rate.[11]

Ticlopidine and clopidogrel

Ticlopidine and clopidogrel are thienopyridines that inhibit the platelet aggregation induced by ADP and, unlike aspirin, do not affect the cyclooxygenase pathway. Both have short half-lives in the circulation and need to be transformed into active metabolites for their antiplatelet effects. They act by blocking an ADP binding site on platelets, which inhibits the expression of the GP IIb/IIIa receptor in the high-affinity configuration that binds fibrinogen and large multimers of von Willebrand factor.[12] Their onset of action is delayed by up to 48–72 hours, and recovery is slow after withdrawal (about 1 week). Large loading doses of clopidogrel are well tolerated and can inhibit platelets more rapidly than ticlopidine.[13]

There are no data concerning the use of ticlopidine or clopidogrel in combination with fibrinolytic agents during the first phases of acute coronary syndrome with ST-segment elevation. An ongoing trial exploring the effectiveness of clopidogrel in the acute phase of MI is the Clopidogrel and Metoprolol in Myocardial Infarction Trial/Second Chinese Cardiac Study (CCS-2), which plans to randomize 40 000 patients according to a 2 × 2 factorial design.[14]

Ridogrel

Ridogrel is a thromboxane A2 synthase inhibitor and a prostaglandin endoperoxide receptor agonist. The randomized trials comparing ridogrel with aspirin as adjuncts to thrombolytic agents have failed to show any advantage for the former, and there are insufficient data to recommend its use in AMI.[15,16]

GP IIb/IIIa antagonists

Rationale for their use in AMI
GP IIb/IIIa receptor inhibitors block the final pathway of any agonist-induced platelet aggregation by inhibiting the binding of fibrinogen to the

receptor of activated platelets in a dose-dependent manner. They also have a disaggregating effect on the white thrombus, which becomes a truly thrombolytic effect on platelet aggregates. This 'dethrombotic' effect is related to various mechanisms: the different affinity constants of GP IIb/IIIa inhibitors and fibrinogen for platelet receptors, the reduced platelet release of plasminogen activator inhibitor-1 (PAI-1), factor XIII and α_2-antiplasmin, the inhibition of factor XIII and α_2-antiplasmin binding to fibrin, and the inhibition of mechanical clot retraction.[17] GP IIb/IIIa inhibitors remove fibrinogen from the fibrin-platelet network because their affinity constant for GP IIb/IIIa receptors is greater than that of fibrinogen. The reduced release of PAI-1 makes the clot more sensitive to fibrinolytic action. As factor XIII and α_2-antiplasmin are important elements in fibrin stabilization, lower concentrations lead to a less organized thrombus that is softer and more easily penetrated by fibrinolytics.

GP IIb/IIIa inhibitors also have antiproliferative, antiinflammatory and anticoagulant activity. The fibrinolysis-induced increase in thrombin concentration not only acts as a prothrombotic stimulus but also reduces fibrinolytic activity by means of the proteolytic activation of thrombin activatable fibrinolysis inhibitor (TAFI) which inhibits fibrinolysis.

It is possible that, in the presence of potent antiplatelet action, the close correlation between activated platelets and the plasma coagulation phase reduces thrombin generation and finally has an efficacious anticoagulant effect.

The efficacy and safety of the combined use of fibrinolytics and GP IIb/IIIa inhibitors have been assessed in numerous animal studies since 1988. The physiopathological rationale underlying the use of this combination is based on the presence of platelet thrombi in necrotic arteries after inefficacious fibrinolytic therapy and the disaggregant action of GP IIb/IIIa inhibitors.[18]

Fibrinolytic therapy involves an increased prothrombotic state related to three mechanisms: (1) the release of thrombin from the fibrin-platelet network (which in turn involves a catalytic action on the fibrinogen that frees new thrombin despite heparin therapy); (2) platelet activation mediated directly by fibrinolytic agents or increased thrombin generation; and (3) the release of plasmin from plasminogen, which activates factor V that, together with Va, Xa and Ca^{2+}, increases the amount of thrombin from prothrombin on the platelet surface (Fig. 3.3).

In *ex vivo* models, the disaggregant action of GP IIb/IIIa inhibitors has been demonstrated by means of aggregometric traces showing that the addition of ADP to platelet-rich serum leads to a rapid increase in transmitted light caused by the rapid formation of platelet macro-aggregates, and that the subsequent addition of abciximab restores the baseline condition of hardly any transmitted light, thus confirming the disaggregation of the macro-aggregates.

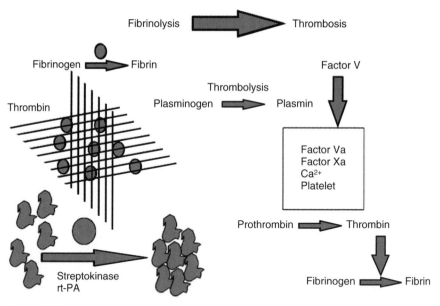

Figure 3.3

The three mechanisms of an increased prothrombotic state during fibrinolytic therapy: (1) the release of thrombin from the fibrin-platelet network; (2) platelet activation due to fibrinolytic agents or an increase in thrombin generation; (3) the release of plasmin from plasminogen that activates factor V which, together with Va, Xa and Ca^{2+}, increases the levels of thrombin from prothrombin.

Studies comparing the efficacy of fibrinolytics alone or in combination with even reduced doses of GP IIb/IIIa inhibitors in animal models with experimental myocardial infarction have demonstrated that the combination leads to a more rapid, complete and stable reperfusion than standard fibrinolytic therapy, without any significant increase in haemorrhagic complications.[19,20]

A new finding that has emerged from the studies of combinations of reduced fibrinolytic doses with glycoprotein inhibitors is the high rate of microcirculation restoration and preservation. In addition to improving the patency of the related necrotic artery, the synergistic action of combined therapy is also shown by the microvessel integrity demonstrated by the rapid normalization of the ST segment.

In TIMI-14, the ST segment normalized in 59% of the patients receiving combined treatment as against 37% of those treated with alteplase alone; among the patients with a TIMI-3 flow, the percentage was also higher in the group that had received alteplase + abciximab (69% vs 44%).[21]

There was a direct linear relationship between ST normalization and mortality, which was about 1% in the patients with complete normalization, a little more than 4% in those with 30–70% resolution and about 5% in the non-normalized subjects.

Antiaggregant and dethrombotic activities transform the platelet-reactive surfaces of complicated plaques into platelet-resistant surfaces, thus leading to a reduction in the distal embolization of platelet aggregates and '*no-reflow*', and the maintenance of microvascular integrity.

Clinical studies

GP IIb/IIIa inhibitors alone. The dethrombotic activity of GP IIb/IIIa inhibitors was explored *in vivo* in the Glycoprotein Receptor Antagonist Patency Evaluation (GRAPE).[22] When given in the emergency room to 60 patients awaiting primary angioplasty without the administration of thrombolytic therapy, abciximab was associated with full reperfusion (TIMI-3 flow grade) in about 20% of the patients, and with TIMI flow grades 2 or 3 in about 40% after a median of 45 min. These figures are higher than those in primary angioplasty trials without such pretreatment.

GP IIb/IIIa inhibitors combined with full doses of fibrinolytics. The first pilot clinical study evaluating the use of GP IIb/IIIa inhibitors during fibrinolytic therapy was the Thrombolysis and Angioplasty in Myocardial Infarction study (TAMI-8). This 'safety' study showed that, when administered at scaled doses and at different times (between 3 and 15 hours after the start of thrombolytic therapy), abciximab did not lead to a greater frequency of haemorrhagic complications when combined with standard tissue plasminogen activator (t-PA) and heparin doses. Furthermore, there was an increase in the percentage of coronary artery patency at the time of discharge (probably as a result of a reduction in reocclusions) and a low frequency of ischaemic events in the patients treated with high doses.[23]

The IMPACT-AMI trial subsequently evaluated the use of different doses of eptifibatide combined with t-PA, aspirin and heparin. The patients treated with high-dose Integrilin and standard-dose t-PA showed a higher percentage of reperfusion (TIMI-3 flow), a lower incidence of reocclusion at follow-up angiography and a 43% reduction in the mean tiime to ST-segment normalization in comparison with the control group.[24]

The combination of eptifibatide and streptokinase was tested in a double-blind, placebo-controlled pilot study whose design was similar to that of IMPACT-AMI. There were no significant between-group differences in TIMI-3 flow percentages, but the incidence of haemorrhagic complications was higher in the patients treated with eptifibatide, and the high-dose arm was abandoned because of excess mortality.[25]

The Platelet Aggregation Receptor Antagonist Dose Investigation and reperfusion Gain in Myocardial Infarction (PARADIGM) dose-exploration study evaluated the combination of lamifiban with t-PA or streptokinase in 353 patients. As assessed by means of ST-segment monitoring, the frequency, speed and stability of the reperfusion of the necrotic artery were greater in the group treated with t-PA and lamifiban, without any significant increase in haemorrhagic complications.[26]

Cumulative analysis of these studies shows that the combination of fibrinolytics and GP IIb/IIIa inhibitors increases the speed and the percentage of complete reperfusion indicated by angiographic and continuous ST-segment monitoring data. However, the study populations were too small and selected (patients at a low stroke of risk) to allow the results to be extrapolated to the general population.

GP IIb/IIIa inhibitors combined with reduced doses of fibrinolytics. The improved reperfusion obtained by combining GPIIb/IIIa inhibitors with low fibrinolytic doses in experimental animal studies, and the risk of haemorrhagic complications when standard fibrinolytic doses are used, led to phase II dose-finding and dose-confirmation clinical trials of combinations including reduced fibrinolytic doses.

The already completed Thrombolysis In Myocardial Infarction (TIMI-14) trial and GUSTO-V pilot study—Strategies for Patency Enhancement in the Emergency Department (SPEED), and in the INTegrilin and Reduced dose Of thrombolytic in Acute Myocardial Infarction (INTRO-AMI) trial, are three international randomized studies with complex designs aimed at identifying the most promising approach for phase III testing.

In TIMI-14, patients with myocardial infarction and ST-segment elevation admitted to hospital within 12 hours of symptom onset were treated with aspirin and randomized to one of 14 different pharmacological regimens: full-dose accelerated alteplase, abciximab alone or one of 12 therapeutic regimens combined with different strategies of abciximab and heparin administration (four with scalar doses of streptokinase and eight with scalar doses of alteplase). The primary end-point was the angiographic evaluation after 90 min; the secondary end-points were the adverse events occurring during hospitalization and during the course of the 30 days' follow-up. Abciximab combined with reduced doses of alteplase and heparin increased TIMI-3 flow in comparison with a standard fibrinolytic dose. The most efficacious combination was abciximab plus 50 mg of alteplase infused over 60 min, which increased the incidence of a related necrotic artery in comparison with alteplase alone from 43% to 72% after 60 min and from 62% to 77% after 90 min. Combined abciximab and alteplase therapy did not increase the risk of haemorrhage, whereas the combination of abciximab and streptokinase led to an unacceptably high risk.[27] The thrombolytic effect of abciximab was confirmed in the patients receiving abciximab alone, in 32% of whom the TIMI-3 flow documented in the related necrotic artery was the same as that obtained with streptokinase in TIMI-1 and GUSTO-I.

The SPEED trial enrolled patients with myocardial infarction and ST-segment elevation within 6 hours of the onset of symptoms, and compared treatment with abciximab alone and in combination with five different reteplase regimens (at scalar doses, or as single or double boluses). All of the patients also received aspirin and low-dose heparin. The primary end-point was the evaluation of TIMI-3 flow in the related necrotic artery after 60 min; the secondary end-points were the major cardiac events of death or reinfarction, recurrent ischaemia requiring revascularization, and haemorrhagic complications after 30 days. The therapeutic regimen that guaranteed the greatest percentage of early and complete reperfusion was the combination of abciximab with a double (5 U + 5 U) reteplase bolus, which led to a 62% incidence of TIMI-3 flow after 60 min. The percentage of haemorrhagic complications was similar in the various groups, and similar to the percentages reported in other studies.[28]

The aim of the INTRO-AMI trial was to evaluate the efficacy of different doses of eptifibatide combined with reduced doses of alteplase (rt-PA). The primary end-point was TIMI-3 flow after 60 min, and the secondary end-points are ST-segment resolution after 180 min and TIMI-3 flow after 90 min. The first phase of the study indicated that the most efficacious treatment for obtaining higher TIMI-3 flow percentages (65% at 60 min and 78% at 90 min) was the combination of various doses of eptifibatide with half the standard dose of rt-PA (a 15 mg bolus followed by a 1 hour 35 mg infusion). The dose-confirmation phase did not show such impressive patency rates (56% at 60 min and 62% at 90 min) although were better than obtained from rt-PA alone (40% and 54%, respectively, at 60 min and 90 min). The improved patency was associated with a slight increase in bleeding, although this was not statistically significant.

GUSTO-V (16 588 patients) was the first phase III study comparing the most promising combination of abciximab and reteplase indicated by the SPEED trial (a double bolus of r-PA 5 U + 5 U and low-dose heparin adjusted on the basis of body weight) with the conventional r-PA double bolus dose plus standard dose heparin. Total 30 day mortality (the primary end-point) was similar in the combination and standard treatment groups (5.6% vs 5.9%: OR 0.95; $p = 0.43$), and there was no difference in the incidence of intracranial haemorrhage or non-fatal cerebrovascular accidents. The percentages of almost all of the complications of myocardial infarction, reinfarction, recurrent ischaemia and the need for urgent revascularization were significantly lower in the patients receiving the combined therapy, but they also experienced a higher number of haemorrhagic complications and episodes of thrombocytopenia.[29] The 1 year results presented at the XIVth World Congress of Cardiology showed no difference in the rate of mortality, which was 8.38% in both groups. No subgroup showed a significant mortality benefit with the combination, although there were slight trends toward greater benefit in diabetic patients and those with anterior myocardial infarction.

The ASSENT (Assessment of the Safety and Efficacy of a New Thrombolytic) 3 trial tested full-dose tenecteplase (TNK-rt-PA) plus enoxaparin, half-dose TNK-rt-PA with weight-adjusted low-dose unfractionated heparin (UFH) infusion and abciximab, and standard treatment with full-dose TNK-rt-PA with weight-adjusted UFH infusion for 48 hours.

The trial randomized 6095 patients within 6 hours of the onset of an acute myocardial infarction to one of the three regimens: the combination of reduced-dose TNK-rt-PA and abciximab was associated with similar 30 day mortality to that of full-dose TNK-rt-PA and UFH or enoxaparin (6.6% vs 6.0% vs 5.4%, respectively, $p = 0.25$). The primary composite end-points (30 day mortality, in-hospital reinfarction or in-hospital refractory ischaemia) were reached in 11.4% of the patients in the enoxaparin group, 11.1% in the abciximab group and 15.4% in the standard treatment group ($p = 0.0001$).

Full-dose TNK-rt-PA with enoxaparin and half-dose lytic plus abciximab and UFH both reduced ischaemic events in comparison with standard treatment using full-dose lytic with heparin, but these benefits were obtained at the cost of a higher rate of bleeding complications particularly in the abciximab group.[30]

The results of these two large-scale trials confirm that the combination of a low dose of a fibrinolytic plus glycoprotein inhibitors is an alternative reperfusion strategy, but cannot immediately be applied in the clinical setting because of the increased risk of haemorrhage, especially in the elderly.[31] Future analyses are necessary (particularly the evaluation of 12 month mortality) in order to define the subgroups of patients in whom the combination has definite advantages over standard treatment.

The ENTIRE-TIMI-23 trial was an open-label, phase II angiographic study in which 461 patients were randomized to full-dose TNK-rt-PA or half-dose TNK-rt-PA plus abciximab, and then further randomized to two corresponding regimens of UFH or varying regimens of enoxaparin with and without an initial intravenous bolus. The primary efficacy end-point was TIMI-3 flow at 60 min, which was obtained by approximately 50% of the patients in each group regardless of the lytic regimen used. The patients randomized to combination therapy tended to have higher rates of ST-segment resolution at 180 min than those receiving standard reperfusion (37% standard, 47% TNK-rt-PA with enoxaparin, 51% with UFH, 59% with enoxaparin). As expected from previous experiences, bleeding rates were higher with the combination of half-dose TNK-rt-PA and abciximab, but appeared to be less with the enoxaparin than the UFH combination.[32]

Primary angioplasty
During vascular injury in the setting of mechanical reperfusion by means of primary angioplasty, platelet activation still occurs by other pathways regardless of acetylsalicylic acid (ASA) inhibition. Platelet activation by any pathway is followed by aggregation, which occurs through the only pathway of the GP IIb/IIIa receptor conformational change that allows them to bind fibrinogen, fibronectin and von Willebrand factor. Intuitively, the inhibition of GPIIb/IIIa receptors seems to be essential during percutaneous revascularization for acute myocardial infarction.

Subgroup analysis of the patients with acute myocardial infarction (AMI) undergoing direct or rescue angioplasty in the EPIC, IMPACT-II, RESTORE and GUSTO-III trials revealed a reduction in the 30 day incidence of death, reinfarction or stroke in patients receiving abciximab compared with the patients who did not.[33–36]

The first prospective randomized study on GP IIb/IIIa inhibitors during primary angioplasty was the ReoPro and Primary PTCA Organization and Randomized Trial (RAPPORT). Among the 438 patients enrolled, the 6 month incidence of death, reinfarction or urgent target vessel revascularization was 49% less in those that underwent angioplasty and received abciximab than in those undergoing angioplasty alone (10.6% vs 20.4%, $p = 0.008$). No intracranial haemorrhage occurred in either group, but the incidence of major bleeding (mainly access-site related) was more frequent in the abciximab-treated patients (16.6% vs 9.5%, $p = 0.02$). The increased bleeding was related to significantly higher activated clotting times (ACTs) at the time of angioplasty in the drug-treated patients, and may be easily overcome by lowering heparin doses when adjunctive GP IIb/IIIa antagonists are used.[37]

The role of GP IIb/IIIa antagonism during primary stenting for AMI has been evaluated in various trials: the Munich Randomized Trial, the Abciximab before Direct Angioplasty and Stenting in Myocardial Infarction Regarding Acute and Long-term Follow-up study (ADMIRAL), the Controlled Abciximab and Device Investigation to Lower Late Angioplasty Complications (CADILLAC), and the Stent versus Thrombolysis for Occluded coronary arteries in Patients with Acute Myocardial Infarction (STOPAMI).

In the Munich Randomized Trial, 200 patients were randomized within 48 hours of an AMI to abciximab or standard therapy before stenting. Coronary blood flow velocities, as measured by means of a flow wire, were significantly greater in the abciximab-treated patients than in those receiving heparin alone and, as no differences in per cent residual stenosis were found between the two groups, this improvement was attributed to greater microvascular perfusion.[38]

The ADMIRAL study was the first placebo-controlled trial to evaluate abciximab as an adjunct to primary percutaneous transluminal coronary angioplasty (PTCA) and stenting. It involved 300 AMI patients who all underwent urgent revascularization plus stenting and were randomly assigned to receive either abciximab or placebo before the intervention. At 30 days, 7.3% in the abciximab group and 14.7% in the placebo group had reached the combined primary end-point of death, reinfarction and urgent target vessel revascularization (TVR). This benefit was maintained at 6 months, by which time the composite end-point had occurred in 16% of the placebo group and 8% of the abciximab group. The rate of major bleeding was similar between the groups, although abciximab was associated with an increased incidence of minor bleeding. About 11% of the

ADMIRAL patients received abciximab or placebo in a mobile intensive care unit an average of 2.8 hours after symptom onset and 1.2 hours earlier than the rest of the study population. They showed a significantly higher rate of pre-intervention TIMI-3 flow than the rest of the abciximab cohort (31.2% vs 12.7%, $p < 0.001$) and a trend towards a higher rate of TIMI-3 flow at 24 hours. However, the small number of early treated patients does not allow any conclusion to be drawn.[39]

CADILLAC enrolled 2665 AMI patients within 12 hours of the infarction, who were randomized to four treatment groups: angioplasty alone; angioplasty plus abciximab; stenting alone; and stenting plus abciximab after angiographic coronarography if they had large enough arteries and appropriate lesions. The primary end-point was the 6 month rate of major adverse clinical events (MACE), which included the composite incidence of death, reinfarction, disabling stroke, or the need for a repeat procedure on the basis of ischaemia. Unlike in previous studies of GP IIb/IIIa antagonism in AMI, there was no significant improvement in outcome with abciximab, although it did tend to improve outcome and slightly decrease mortality in PTCA patients. The 6 month MACE rate was virtually the same in the two stent groups: 10.9% in those receiving a stent alone; 10.8% in those also receiving abciximab.

The discordance between the results of this and previous studies is presumably due to differences in study design (inclusion criteria, such as angiographic selection; the timing of drug administration) and in the end-point.[40]

In the STOPAMI study 140 patients were randomly assigned to receive a stent plus abciximab versus intravenous alteplase. The primary end-point (i.e. the degree of myocardial salvage determined by means of serial scintigraphic studies using technetium Tc 99 m sestamibi) was greater in the patients undergoing stenting with GP IIb/IIIa inhibition. The number of patients reaching the combined end-point of death, reinfarction or stroke after 6 months was also lower in the stent plus abciximab group (8.5% vs 23.2%).[41]

Facilitated angioplasty

Facilitated angioplasty has become more widespread since the publication of the results of intervention studies showing a reduction in major cardiac complications in AMI patients undergoing revascularization procedures after the combined administration of fibrinolytics and glycoprotein inhibitors in comparison with those administered fibrinolysis alone.[33] It is thought that the 'facilitation' is substantially due to two factors: reduced stenosis and the 'passivation' of platelet-reactive surfaces at the time of angioplasty. The antiplatelet and dethrombotic action of glycoprotein inhibitors reduces the stenosis by blocking the growth and promoting the lysis of the intracoronary thrombus, thus favouring the creation of a lumen favourable for revascularization; it also reduces the risk of early thrombotic reocclusion and distal platelet embolization by creating optimal rheological conditions.

Studies in which glycoprotein inhibitors have been combined with the use of a stent have also revealed a positive synergism in reducing major cardiac events. Although referring to elective revascularization procedures rather than situations of acute myocardial infarction with ST-segment elevation, this is clearly shown by the data coming from the EPISTENT (Evaluation of Platelet IIb/IIIa Inhibitor for STENTing),[42] and ESPRIT (Enhanced Suppression of the Platelet IIb/IIIa Receptor with Integrilin Therapy) studies.[43] During the acute phase, the stent reduces the risk of occlusion due to mechanical causes as a result of its greater control over dissections and the fact that it establishes a larger vessel lumen, whereas GP IIb/IIIa inhibitors prevent acute thrombotic complications by ensuring the 'passivation' of the plaque and the surfaces of the prosthesis.

During the angiographic evaluation forming part of the protocol of the SPEED study, 61% of the patients underwent angioplasty an average of 62 min after the start of reperfusion therapy. The success rate was very high in the patients receiving combined therapy, varying from 80% to 90% in the different groups with no significant difference between them. Furthermore, angioplasty was used less frequently in the patients who had received a double bolus of abciximab combined with reteplase because they had the highest TIMI-3 flow percentage at the initial angiographic examination (86% after 90 min).[28] Combined therapy therefore guaranteed a high rate of success in patients who could not undergo percutaneous revascularization for anatomical reasons, as well as in those who were treated with angioplasty.

Prospective large-scale studies are needed to evaluate the efficacy and safety of early triple combination reperfusion therapy for facilitated coronary angioplasty.

Chronic phase of myocardial infarction

Aspirin

Monotherapy alone

In the Antiplatelet Trialist's Collaboration study of 20 543 patients, there was a 26% relative reduction in death or myocardial infarction (MI) in the patients treated with aspirin in comparison with those treated with placebo (10.6% vs 14.4%; $p < 0.001$).[44] The Antiplatelet Trialist's Collaboration overview of prolonged (mainly aspirin) antiplatelet therapy in about 70 000 high-risk patients participating in 145 trials showed a risk reduction of 30% in non-fatal MI, 30% in non-fatal stroke and 17% in vascular death. It is estimated that aspirin prevents 35–40 occurrences of the thrombotic complications of atherosclerotic complications per 1000 treated patients. The daily doses used in these trials were 500–1500 mg, 160–325 mg and 75–150 mg.

The adverse effects of aspirin are primarily related to (particularly gastrointestinal) bleeding, although this is less frequent at low doses of 80–160 mg/day and with the enteric-coated form. In long-term management, patients should continue to receive aspirin for an indefinite period after acute MI for purposes of secondary prevention.

Monotherapy vs anticoagulation therapy
Some studies have investigated whether aspirin alone offers a benefit over anticoagulation therapy in long-term secondary prevention.

The German-Austrian Reinfarction Study and the French Enquéte de Prévention Secondaire de l'Infarctus du Myocard (EPSIM) study were long-term trials performed during the chronic phase of MI that compared oral anticoagulants with aspirin in patients who had not undergone thrombolytic therapy. After, respectively, 24 and 29 months of follow-up, the groups treated with aspirin 1.5 g/day showed a trend towards a reduction in coronary death but an increased rate of peptic ulcer.[45,46]

A meta-analysis of the few small trials comparing moderate-to-high intensity anticoagulation versus aspirin did not demonstrate any difference in efficacy, whereas the rate of bleeding was lower with aspirin.[47]

Monotherapy vs combination therapy
The Coumadin, Aspirin Reinfarction Study (CARS) was a randomized double-blind trial involving 8803 patients enrolled 3–21 days after MI who received aspirin 160 mg, or warfarin 1 mg plus aspirin 80 mg, or warfarin 3 mg plus aspirin 80 mg. After 14 months of follow-up, reinfarction, non-fatal ischaemic stroke or cardiovascular death had occurred in, respectively, 8.6%, 8.8% and 8.4% of the patients. Low fixed-dose warfarin (1 mg or 3 mg) combined with low-dose aspirin (80 mg) did not provide any additional clinical benefit over aspirin 160 mg alone. The results suggested that warfarin therapy is effective in short-term secondary prevention only at an international normalization ratio (INR) of 2–3.5.[48]

The Combination Hemotherapy and Mortality Prevention (CHAMP) trial was a randomized multicentre trial involving 5059 patients enrolled up to 14 days after acute myocardial infarction (AMI) who received aspirin 160 mg, or warfarin, to maintain an INR of 1.5–2.5 plus aspirin 80 mg. Approximately 40% of the patients had suffered a Q-wave infarction, 30% of whom had received thrombolytic therapy. After 2.75 years of follow-up, the rates of death, non-fatal reinfarction, stroke, and cerebral and fatal bleeding were similar in the two groups. Major bleeding requiring transfusions occurred in 1.9% of the patients treated with aspirin alone and 3.4% of those in the anticoagulant plus aspirin group.[49]

The data of the second Warfarin-Aspirin Re-Infarction Study (WARIS II) presented at the XXIII Congress of the European Society of Cardiology suggest that the combination of warfarin and aspirin is superior to either agent alone in reducing death and recurrent events after MI. Between January 1994 and June 1998, 3630 patients treated for MI were randomized in an open-label fashion to aspirin alone (160 mg/day), warfarin alone with a target INR of 2.8–4.2, or a combination of both agents at lower doses (aspirin 75 mg/day and warfarin with a target INR of 2.0–2.5), and followed for a mean of about 4 years. Q-wave infarction had occurred in 59% of the cases, and 54% had received thrombolytic therapy. The primary end-point (the rate of the first occurrence of the composite outcome of death from any cause, non-fatal reinfarction and thromboembolic stroke) was 20% in the aspirin group, 16.7% in the warfarin group and 15% in the combination group, with a 29% relative risk reduction between the aspirin and the combination group. However, the benefit of the combination arm over warfarin alone did not reach statistical significance (OR 0.88; 95% CI 0.72–1.07, $p = 0.20$). Major and minor bleedings were more frequent in the warfarin (major 0.58%/year; minor 2.16%/year) and combination arms (major 0.52%/year; minor 2.75%/year) than in the aspirin arm (major 0.15%/year; minor 0.81%/year), but the absolute numbers were very low.[50,51]

These data are very important, but any change in clinical practice requires more than one trial reporting the same results. It is also necessary to remember that long-term aspirin therapy is simple, safe and inexpensive. It remains to be seen how the results of WARIS II can be integrated with the CURE data and the possible association of clopidogrel with an oral anticoagulant.

The results of these trials led to the current guidelines suggesting that an initial aspirin dose of 160–325 mg/day should be given as soon as possible, in the early management of all patients with a suspected acute AMI. After the first 24 hours, when the embolic risk is low, the patients with AMI should continue to receive aspirin 80–325 mg/day indefinitely. In the presence of an allergy to aspirin, other antiplatelet agents must be considered. The patients at increased embolic risk (AMI complicated by severe left ventricular dysfunction, chronic heart failure, previous embolism, atrial fibrillation, or 2D-echocardiographic evidence of mural thrombosis) should receive warfarin for at least 6 months after MI.

Clopidogrel

There are no trials comparing the role of ticlopidine with that of aspirin or other antiplatelet agents in the prevention of cardiovascular death or reinfarction in the chronic phase after myocardial infarction.

Clopidogrel was evaluated in the Clopidogrel Versus Aspirin in Patients at Risk of Ischaemic Events (CAPRIE)[52] and CURE trials.[53] In the CAPRIE trial, a *post hoc* analysis of the 8446 patients with a history of MI revealed a non-significant risk reduction of 7.4% in the primary end-point of death, new MI or vascular death in the clopidogrel-treated patients; no fatal complications were reported. The combination of clopidogrel with aspirin has synergistic thrombosis-inhibiting effects.

CURE was a randomized, double-blind, parallel-group study in which 12 562 patients with acute coronary syndrome (ACS) or non-Q-wave MI received aspirin 75–325 mg and were then randomly assigned to clopido-grel (300 mg load followed by 75 mg daily) or placebo for between three months and one year. There was a 20% relative risk reduction in the primary end-point ($p = 0.00005$), due to a 23% relative reduction in MI. Interestingly, there was a trend towards a reduction in the risk of stroke, with no excess in intracranial bleeding, and also a trend towards a reduc-tion in the risk of cardiovascular (CV) death. The primary end-point was a composite of CV death, MI or stroke. The benefits of clopidogrel accrued very early, with a 20% relative reduction by the end of the first day. When severe ischaemia was added to the analysis, there was a statistically significant 33% relative risk reduction by the end of the first day (149 vs 100 events). A 34% excess of major bleeding was observed (3.6% vs 2.7% in the placebo group; $p = 0.003$), but no significant excess of life-threatening bleeding (2.1% vs 1.8%, $p = 0.27$). Minor bleedings were more frequent in the clopidogrel arm (1.6% vs 1.0%, $p < 0.0001$). No cases of neutropenia or thrombotic thrombocytopenic purpura were reported.

Clopidogrel has a more favourable side-effect profile than ticlopidine and is therefore preferable in patients who are resistant or hypersensitive to aspirin, or in whom aspirin is otherwise contraindicated.

The safety and a lower rate of serious side effects with the combination of aspirin plus clopidogrel in comparison with aspirin plus ticlopidine was reported in the Clopidogrel Aspirin Stent International Cooperative Study (CLASSIC).[13]

Oral GP IIb/IIIa antagonists

There are no trials of oral GP IIb/IIIa inhibitors in patients with acute coro-nary syndrome (ACS) with ST-segment elevation. The only trial involved coronary intervention and non-ST-segment elevation. The fact that the intravenous administration of GP IIb/IIIa antagonists reduces the death rate and MI in these situations aroused great interest in the possibility that oral GP IIb/IIIa inhibitors may offer a benefit in the long-term treat-ment of an episode after an acute coronary syndrome. Xemilofiban was studied in the EXCITE trial, orbofiban in the OPUS-TIMI-16 trial and sibrafiban in the SYMPHONY I and SYMPHONY II trials. When all four trials are taken together, oral GP IIb/IIIa blockers are associated with a highly significant 35% increase in mortality.[54–56]

Recent studies have suggested a number of pathophysiological, pharmacokinetic and pharmacodynamic explanations for the apparent toxicity of the oral GP IIb/IIIa agents tested so far, including their prothrombotic activity, pro-inflammatory action, short half-life, high peak-trough ratio, low receptor affinity and preference for binding to the active rather than the inactive receptor.

References

1. Mac Isaac AI, Thomas EJ. Toward the quiescent plaque. J Am Coll Cardiol 1993; **22**: 1128–41.

2. Falk E, Shah PK, Fuster V. Coronary plaque disruption. Circulation 1995; **92**:657–71.

3. Fernandez-Ortiz A, Badimon JJ, Falk E et al. Characterization of the relative thrombogenecity of atherosclerotic plaque components: implication for plaque rupture. J Am Coll Cardiol 1994; **23**:1562–9.

4. Nurden AT, Bihour C, Macchi L et al. Platelet activation in thrombotic disorders. Nouv Rev Fr Hematol 1993; **35**:67–71.

5. Fleming TG. Von Willebrand factor: its function and its measurement in the laboratory. Br J Biomed Sci 1995; **52**:50–7.

6. Shah PK. Pathophysiology of plaque rupture and the concept of plaque stabilization. Cardiol Clin 1996; **14**:17–29.

7. Ofosu FA, Sie P, Modi GJ et al. The inhibition of thrombin-dependent positive feedback reactions is critical to the expression of the anticoagulant effect of heparin. Biochem J 1987; **243**: 579.

8. Shah PK. New insights into the pathogenesis and prevention of acute coronary syndromes. Am J Cardiol 1997; **79**:17–23.

9. ISIS-2 investigators. Randomised trial of intravenous streptokinase, oral aspirin, both, or neither among 17,187 cases of suspected acute myocardial infarction: ISIS-2 (Second International Study of Infarct Survival) Collaborative Group. Lancet 1988; **2**:349–60.

10. Veen G, Meyer A, Verheugt FW et al. Culprit lesion morphology and stenosis severity in the prediction of reocclusion after coronary thrombolysis: angiographic results of the APRICOT study. Antithrombotics in the Prevention of Reocclusion in Coronary Thrombolysis. J Am Coll Cardiol 1993; **22**:1755–62.

11. Julian DG, Chamberlain DA, Pocock SJ et al. A comparison of aspirin and anticoagulation following thrombolysis for myocardial infarction (the AFTER study): a multicentre unblinded randomised clinical trial. BMJ 1996; **313**:1429–31.

12. Sharis PJ, Cannon CP, Loscalzo J. The antiplatelet effects of ticlopidine and clopidogrel. Ann Intern Med 1998; **129**:394–405.

13. The CLASSIC Study: Clopidogrel + ASA vs. Ticlopidin + ASA in patients with stents. Internist (Berlin) 1999; **40**(suppl 5: Clopidogrel):1–4.

14. CCS-2. Second Chinese Cardiac Study Collaborative Group. Rationale, design and organization of the Second Chinese Cardiac Study: a randomized

trial of clopidogrel plus aspirin, and of metoprolol, among patients with suspected acute myocardial infarction. Second Chinese Cardiac Study (CCS-2) Collaborative Group. J Cardiovasc Risk 2000; **7**:435–41.

15. Tranchesi B, Pileggi F, Vercammen E, Van de Werf F, Verstraete M. Ridogrel does not increase the speed and rate of coronary recanalization in patients with myocardial infarction treated with alteplase and heparin. Eur Heart J 1994; **15**: 660–4.

16. RAPT Randomized trial of ridogrel, a combined thromboxane A2 synthase inhibitor and thromboxane A2/prostaglandin endoperoxide receptor antagonist, versus aspirin as adjunct to thrombolysis in patients with acute myocardial infarction. The Ridogrel Versus Aspirin Patency Trial (RAPT). Circulation 1994; **89**:588–95.

17. Coller BS Augmentation of thrombolysis with antiplatelet drugs. Overview. Coron Arter Dis 1995; **6**:911–14.

18. Falk E. Thrombosis in unstable angina: pathologic aspects. Cardiovasc Clin 1987; **18**:137–49.

19. Yasuda T, Gold HK, Leinbach RC et al. Lysis of plasminogen activator-resistant platelet-rich coronary artery thrombus with combined bolus injection of recombinant tissue-type plasminogen activator and antiplatelet GPIIb/IIIa antibody. J Am Coll Cardiol 1990; **16**:1728–35.

20. Mickelson JK, Simpson PJ, Cronin M et al. Antiplatelet antibody [7E3 F(ab')2] prevents rethrombosis after recombinant tissue-type plasminogen activator-induced coronary artery thrombolysis in a canine model. Circulation 1990; **81**:617–27.

21. de Lemons JA, Antman EM, Gibson M et al. Abciximab improves both epicardial flow and myocardial reperfusion in ST-elevation myocardial infarction. Observations from the TIMI 14 trial. Circulation 2000; **101**: 239–43.

22. van den Merkhof LF, Zijlstra F, Olsson H et al. Abciximab in the treatment of acute myocardial infarction eligible for primary percutaneous transluminal coronary angioplasty. Results of the Glycoprotein Receptor Antagonist Patency Evaluation (GRAPE) pilot study. J Am Coll Cardiol 1999; **33**(6):1528–32.

23. Kleiman NS, Ohamn EM, Califf RM et al. Profound inhibition of platelet aggregation with monoclonal antibody 7E3 Fab after thrombolytic therapy: results of the Thrombolysis and Angioplasty in Myocardial Infarction (TAMI) 8 pilot study. J Am Coll Cardiol 1993; **22**:381–9.

24. Ohman EM, Leiman NS, Gacioch G et al. for the IMPACT-AMI Investigators. Combined accelerated tissue-plasminogen activator and platelet glycoprotein IIb/IIIa integrin receptor blockade with Integrilin in acute myocardial infarction. Circulation 1997; **95**:846–54.

25. Ronner E, van Kesteren HAM, Zijnen P et al. Combined therapy with streptokinase and Integrilin. J Am Coll Cardiol 1998; **31**:191A (Abstract).

26. PARADIGM investigators. Combining thrombolysis with the platelet glycoprotein IIb/IIIa inhibitor lamifiban: results of the Platelet Aggregation Receptor Antagonist Dose Investigation and reperfusion Gain in Myocardial Infarction (PARADIGM) trial. J Am Coll Cardiol 1998; **32**: 2003–10.

27. Antman EM, Giugliano RP, Gibson CM et al. for the Thrombolysis in Myocardial Infarction (TIMI) 14 Investigators. Abciximab facilitates the rate and extent of thrombolysis: results of Thrombolysis in Myocardial Infarction (TIMI) 14 trial. Circulation 1999; **99**:2720–32.

28. SPEED investigators trial of abciximab with and without low-dose reteplase for acute myocardial infarction. Strategies for Patency Enhancement in the Emergency Department (SPEED) Group. Circulation 2000; **101**:2788–94.

29. The GUSTO-V investigators. Reperfusion therapy for acute myocardial infarction with fibrinolytic therapy or combination reduced fibrinolytic therapy and platelet glycoprotein IIb/IIIa inhibition: the GUSTO-V randomised trial. Lancet 2001; **357**:1905–14.

30. (ASSENT)-3 investigators. The Assessment of the Safety and Efficacy of a New Thrombolytic Regimen. Efficacy and safety of tenecteplase in combination with enoxaparin, abciximab, or unfractionated heparin: the ASSENT-3 randomised trial in acute myocardial infarction. Lancet 2001; **358**:605–13.

31. Freek W Verheugt. Risk and benefit of half-dose lytic plus abciximab versus lytic alone for ST-elevation myocardial infarction: a meta-analysis. American College of Cardiology Abstracts 2002; **39**:204B, 3162.

32. Antman EM, Louwerenburg HW, Baars HF et al. for the ENTIRE-Thrombolysis in Myocardial Infarction (TIMI) 23 Investigators. Enoxaparin as adjunctive antithrombin therapy for ST-elevation myocardial infarction. Results of the ENTIRE-TIMI 23 trial. Circulation 2002; **105**:1642–9.

33. Lefkovits J, Ivanhoe RJ, Califf RM et al. Effects of platelet glycoprotein IIb/IIIa receptor blockade by a chimeric monoclonal antibody (abciximab) on acute and six-month outcomes after percutaneous transluminal coronary angioplasty for acute myocardial infarction. EPIC investigators. Am J Cardiol 1996; **77**:1045–51.

34. IMPACT-II investigators. Randomised placebo-controlled trial of effect of eptifibatide on complications of percutaneous coronary intervention: IMPACT-II. Integrilin to Minimise Platelet Aggregation and Coronary Thrombosis-II. Lancet 1997; **349**:1422–8.

35. RESTORE investigators. Effects of platelet glycoprotein IIb/IIIa blockade with tirofiban on adverse cardiac events in patients with unstable angina or acute myocardial infarction undergoing coronary angioplasty. Randomized Efficacy Study of Tirofiban for Outcomes and REstenosis. Circulation 1997; **96**:1445–53.

36. Grantham JA, Hasdai D, Kopecky SL, Holmes DR. Platelet glycoprotein IIb/IIIa inhibition during PTCA for acute MI. J Am Coll Cardiol 1998; **31**:231A (Abstract).

37. Brener SJ, Barr LA, Burchenal JEB et al. for the RAPPORT investigators. A randomized, placebo-controlled trial of platelet glycoprotein IIb/IIIa blockade with primary angioplasty for acute myocardial infarction. Circulation 1998; **98**:734–41.

38. Schomig A, Neumann FJ, Walter H et al. Coronary stent placement in patients with acute myocardial infarction: comparison of clinical and angiographic outcome after randomization to antiplatelet or anticoagulant

therapy. J Am Coll Cardiol 1997; **29**:28–34.

39. Montalescot G, Barragan P, Wittenberg O et al. ADMIRAL Investigators. Abciximab before Direct Angioplasty and Stenting in Myocardial Infarction Regarding Acute and Long-Term Follow-up. N Engl J Med 2001 **344**: 1895–903.

40. Stone GW, Grines CL, Cox DA et al. Comparison of angioplasty with stenting, with or without abciximab, in acute myocardial infarction. N Engl J Med 2002; **346**:957–66.

41. Schömig A, Kastrati A, Dirschinger J et al. For the Stent versus Thrombolysis for Occluded Coronary Arteries in Patients with Acute Myocardial Infarction Study Investigators. Coronary stenting plus platelet glycoprotein IIb/IIa blockade compared with tissue plasminogen activator in acute myocardial infarction. N Engl J Med 2000; **343**:385–91.

42. EPISTENT investigators. Randomised placebo-controlled and balloon-angioplasty-controlled trial to assess safety of coronary stenting with use of platelet glycoprotein-IIb/IIIa blockade. Evaluation of Platelet IIb/IIIa Inhibitor for Stenting. Lancet 1998; **352**:87–92.

43. O'Shea JC, Hafley GE, Greenberg S et al. Platelet glycoprotein IIb/IIIa integrin blockade with eptifibatide in coronary stent intervention: the ESPRIT trial: a randomized controlled trial. JAMA 2001; **285**:2468–73.

44. Antiplatelet Trialists' Collaboration. Collaborative overview of randomised trials of antiplatelet therapy: III. Reduction in venous thrombosis and pulmonary embolism by antiplatelet prophylaxis among surgical and medical patients. BMJ 1994; **308**:235–46.

45. Breddin D, Loew D, Lechner K et al. The German-Austrian Aspirin trial: a comparison of acetylsalicylic acid, placebo and phenprocoumon in secondary prevention of myocardial infarction. Circulation 1980; **62**:V63–V72.

46. The EPSIM Research Group. A controlled comparison of aspirin and oral anticoagulants in prevention of death after myocardial infarction. N Engl J Med 1982; **307**:701–8.

47. Anand SS, Yusuf S. Oral anticoagulant therapy in patients with coronary artery disease: a meta-analysis. JAMA 1999; **282**: 2058–67.

48. Coumadin, Aspirin, Reinfarction Study (CARS) investigators. Randomized, double-blind trial of fixed low dose warfarin with aspirin after myocardial infarction. Lancet 1997; **350**:389–96.

49. Fiore LD, Ezekowitz MD, Brophy MT, Lu D, Sacco J, Peduzzi P. Department of Veterans Affairs Cooperative Studies Program Clinical Trial comparing combined warfarin and aspirin with aspirin alone in survivors of acute myocardial infarction: primary results of the CHAMP study. Circulation 2002; **105**: 557–63.

50. Arnesen H. Second Warfarin-Aspirin Re-Infarction Study (WARIS II). XXIII Congress of the European Society of Cardiology 2001.

51. Coletta AP, Cleland JG. Clinical trials update: highlights of the scientific sessions of the XXIII Congress of the European Society of Cardiology—WARIS II, ESCAMI, PAFAC, RITZ-1 and TIME. Eur J Heart Fail 2001; **3**:747–50.

52. CAPRIE Steering Committee. A randomised, blinded, trial of clopidogrel versus aspirin in

patients at risk of ischaemic events (CAPRIE). Lancet 1996; **348**:1329–39.

53. CURE Study investigators. Effects of clopidogrel in addition to aspirin in patients with non ST-elevation acute coronary syndromes. N Engl J Med 2001; **345**:494–502.

54. O'Neill WW, Serruys P, Knudtson M et al. Long-term treatment with a platelet glycoprotein-receptor antagonist after percutaneous coronary revascularization. EXCITE Trial Investigators. Evaluation of Oral Xemilofiban in Controlling Thrombotic Events. N Engl J Med 2000; **342**:1316.

55. Cannon CP, McCabe CH, Wilcox RG et al. Oral glycoprotein IIb/IIIa inhibition with orbofiban in patients with unstable coronary syndromes (OPUS-TIMI 16) trial. Circulation 2000; **102**:149–56.

56. SYMPHONY investigators. Comparison of sibrafiban with aspirin for prevention of cardiovascular events after acute coronary syndromes: a randomised trial. Sibrafiban versus Aspirin to Yield Maximum Protection from Ischemic Heart Events Post-acute Coronary Syndromes. Lancet 2000; **355**:337–45.

4

Anticoagulants as adjunctive therapy in fibrinolysis for acute myocardial infarction

Marc A Brouwer and Freek W A Verheugt

Introduction

With the knowledge that acute thrombotic occlusion of a major epicardial coronary artery is the most common pathophysiological mechanism in acute ST-segment elevation myocardial infarction, fibrinolytic therapy has become standard therapy. It is easy to administer and, in contrast to mechanical reperfusion therapy by primary angioplasty, it is widely available. The costs are moderate and the benefit of in-hospital treatment is important: approximately 20 lives saved per 1000 treated patients.[1] Especially in very early, and preferably, pre-hospital treatment an additional 18 lives per 1000 can be saved.[2] Outcome after fibrinolytic therapy can be improved by adjuvant antiplatelet therapy, such as aspirin, and very likely, also by anticoagulant treatment.[3]

Current anticoagulant therapy can be divided in parenteral and oral treatment. Parenteral therapy is mainly aimed at the inhibition of thrombin activity; oral treatment interferes with the formation of coagulation factors involved in thrombin generation and the propagation of coronary thrombosis.

Antithrombin therapy in fibrinolysis

Since fibrinolytic therapy is accompanied by intensive thrombin generation and activation, immediate and continuous adjunctive therapy with intravenous unfractionated heparin is recommended.[3] The effect of heparin is mediated through activation of antithrombin III—so-called indirect thrombin inhibition. Heparin is thought to block the thrombin activity observed in acute coronary thrombosis and counteract thrombin generated by the fibrinolytic treatment. The paradoxical procoagulant state induced by fibrinolytic therapy is considered to be one of the mechanisms in the occurrence of early coronary reocclusion.[4] Yet, a benefit of immediate, concomitant heparinization on early patency and reocclusion after fibrinolytic therapy has never been firmly established in patients treated with aspirin.[3,4] As far as the subsequent 48-hour infusion is concerned, observational data suggest an effect on recurrent ischaemia and clinical reinfarction; a clustering of recurrent ischaemic events has been reported early after discontinuation of anticoagulation therapy.[5]

Both for safety and efficacy, heparin therapy needs close monitoring using the activated partial thromboplastin time (APTT). The level of APTT at 12 hours after lytic therapy has been shown to predict the risk of moderate and severe haemorrhage, and most importantly, the risk of intracranial bleeding.[3,5] Noteworthy, patient-related factors have the strongest relationship with bleeding: (increasing) age, female sex, hypertension and low bodyweight.[6] Lowering the dose of heparin results in a reduction of intracranial haemorrhage without loss of clinical efficacy.[7] In the current guidelines, the recommended dose of heparin has therefore been changed into a bolus of 60 U/kg to a maximum of 4000 U followed by a continuous infusion (12 U/kg/h, maximum 1000 U/h) of at least 48 hours with a target APTT of 50–70 seconds. Earlier and more frequent monitoring—3, 6, 12 and 24 hours after the first dose—constitutes an additional adjustment.[8]

As an alternative, direct thrombin inhibition has been studied extensively in patients undergoing fibrinolytic therapy for acute myocardial infarction. In contrast to indirect thrombin inhibition, direct thrombin inhibitors are also able to inhibit clot-bound thrombin. Moreover, frequent monitoring is not required. In two large clinical trials including over 7000 patients with ST-elevation myocardial infarction, hirudin showed no benefit in mortality and a trend towards lower reinfarction rates as compared to heparin. This is at the expense of increased bleeding.[9,10] The same has been observed recently in a 17 000 patients' trial with the less expensive specific thrombin inhibitor hirulog.[11]

Low molecular weight heparins (LMWHs) have a better bioavailability, induce less platelet activation, and administration can more easily be extended than unfractionated heparin (UFH) because of their subcutaneous administration. In addition to inhibition of thrombin activity, it has a marked impact higher in the coagulation cascade, exerted on factor Xa. Three angiographic trials were performed addressing their impact in conjunction with fibrinolytic therapy. In the placebo-controlled AMI-SK study, LMWH proved effective with respect to early ST resolution and 5 day patency after streptokinase. In conjunction with rt-PA there seemed at least equivalence to UFH (Table 4.1).[12–14] In these studies the LMWH was given as a bolus together with the lytic drug, and continued subcutaneously twice daily until coronary angiographic evaluation.

Interestingly, in ASSENT-PLUS dalteparin reduced reocclusion and reinfarction rates during treatment, whereas 30 day reinfarction rates were similar to patients in the control arm.[12] A subsidiary analysis in HART-II, studying the subset of patients with TIMI-3 flow at 90 min angiography, suggested lower reocclusion rates at 5–7 days: 9% with UFH compared to 3% with enoxaparin ($p = 0.12$).[13] Similar observations have been reported

Table 4.1 New anticoagulants as adjuvants to fibrinolytic therapy for acute myocardial infarction.

Study	Fibrinolytic agent	New anticoagulant	TIMI-3 flow	
			New treatment	UFH
			90 minutes	
HART-II[13]	rt-PA	Enoxaparin	101/191 (53%)	90/189 (48%)
PENTALYSE[15]	rt-PA	Pentasaccharide	148/232 (64%)	57/84 (68%)
			3–5 days	
AMI-SK[14]	SK	Enoxaparin	~178/253 (70%)	~141/243 (58%)[a]
ASSENT-PLUS[12]	rt-PA	Dalteparin	140/202 (69%)	110/176 (63%)

[a] Placebo; $p = 0.01$, numbers are estimates based on the percentages provided in 389 patients with evaluable angiograms.
UFH, unfractionated heparin; rt-PA, recombinant tissue plasminogen activator; SK, streptokinase.

in the PENTALYSE trial, testing pentasaccharide, a specific Xa inhibitor (Table 4.1).[15] In contrast to HART-II, the new antithrombotic regimen was administered longer (5–7 days) than UFH (2–3 days). In the subset of patients without signs of recurrent ischaemia, reocclusion was reduced from 7% on UFH to 0.9% on the pentasaccharide ($p = 0.06$).

To date, two clinical trials have been performed to provide better insight on the safety and efficacy of LMWH as adjunctive therapy. In the ASSENT-3 trial, enoxaparin (i.v. bolus followed by subcutaneous injections twice daily until discharge) has been compared to UFH (bolus followed by infusion for at least 48 hours) as adjunct to the bolus lytic agent tenecteplase (TNK-tPA) in over 4000 patients.[16] The enoxaparin regimen turned out to be superior to UFH on the combined primary endpoint of 30 day mortality, in-hospital reinfarction and reischaemia. This benefit was primarily driven by a reduction in recurrent ischaemic events, and was lost at 1 year follow-up which included out-of-hospital reinfarctions.[17] The early clinical benefit was obtained with a 40% increase in severe bleeding, but not cerebral bleeding. However, in the recently presented ASSENT-3-PLUS study cerebral bleeding was unacceptably increased by bolus enoxaparin (Table 4.2).[18] In this randomized trial, 1639 patients treated with pre-hospitally administered tenecteplase were randomized to a bolus of UFH (followed by in-hospital infusion for at least 48 hours) or a bolus of enoxaparin (followed by in-hospital subcutaneous injections twice daily). Again, the (longer) administration of enoxaparin resulted in lower rates of recurrent ischaemic events. More importantly, however, 12 of the 61 deaths observed on enoxaparin were bleeding-related, as compared to only 3 out of 49 in the control arm.[18]

Thus, current antithrombin therapy following fibrinolytic therapy seems to be optimal with UFH, which is given as a bolus together with the lytic (preferably tenecteplase) and continued for at least 48 hours. Definitive guidelines with respect to the use of LMWHs should be based on more clinical data, especially those on safety. These issues will be studied in the large-scale EXTRACT-TIMI-25 clinical trial, in which age-dependent doses of subcutaneous injections with and without bolus will be compared to UFH bolus plus infusion after lytic therapy with either alteplase, tenecteplase, reteplase or streptokinase.

An alternative therapy following the bolus of UFH, could be subcutaneous administration of enoxaparin until hospital discharge. In view of the above observations that a prolonged regimen of antithrombin therapy is effective, this may reduce in-hospital reocclusion and recurrent ischaemic events.

Oral anticoagulation after myocardial infarction (Table 4.3)

Given the promising results of a prolonged in-hospital regimen of both antiplatelet and antithrombin therapy, oral anticoagulation seems

Table 4.2 Risks of using novel anticoagulant therapy as an adjuvant to fibrinolytic therapy for acute myocardial infarction.

Study	Fibrinolytic agent	New anticoagulant	Cerebral bleeding		
			LMWH		UFH
ASSENT-3[16]	TNK-tPA	Enoxaparin	18/2040 (0.9%)		19/2038 (0.9%)
ASSENT-3PLUS[18]	TNK-tPA	Enoxaparin	18/818 (2.2%)	a	8/827 (1.0%)
Total LMWH			36/2858 (1.3%)	b	27/2863 (0.9%)
			Pentasaccharide		UFH
PENTALYSE[15]	rt-PA	ORG31540/SR9017A	1/241 (0.4%)		0/85 (0.0%)

[a] $p = 0.05$; [b] $p = 0.18$.
LMWH, low molecular weight heparin; UFH, unfractionated heparin; TNK-tPA, tenecteplase; rt-PA, recombinant tissue plasminogen activator.

Table 4.3 Randomized aspirin-controlled studies of oral anticoagulation as an adjuvant to aspirin after acute coronary syndromes.

Study	Year	N	INR target	INR reached	ASA dose (mg)	1° end-point ASA+OAC	1° end-point ASA	RR 95% CI	p-value	Fup (mths)
Angiographic						*% (re)occlusion*				
Williams et al.[25]	1997	57	2.0–2.5	2.0	150	4%	33%	n.a.	0.02[a]	3
APRICOT-2[22]	2002	308	2.0–3.0	2.6	80	15%	28%	0.55 (0.33–0.90)	< 0.02	3
Clinical						*% mortality, (re)MI, stroke*				
CARS[20]	1997	8803	1 mg qd		80 vs 160	8.8%	8.6%	1.03 (0.87–1.22)	0.74	14
			3 mg qd			8.4%		0.95 (0.81–1.12)	0.57	14
CHAMP[21]	2002	5059	1.5–2.5	1.8	80 vs 160	17.6%[b]	17.3%[b]	0.98 (0.87–1.11)	0.76	33
ASPECT-2[23]	2002	668	2.0–2.5	2.4	80	5.0%	9.0%	0.50 (0.27–0.92)	< 0.05	12
OASIS-2[26]	2001	3712	2.0–2.5	np	Not specified	7.6%	8.3%	0.90 (0.72–1.14)	0.40	5
Good compliers		1821				6.1%	8.9%	0.68 (0.48–0.95)	0.02	
Poor compliers		1891				9.0%	7.8%	1.17 (0.86–1.60)	0.33	
WARIS-II[24]	2002	2414	2.0–2.5	2.2	75 vs 160	15.0%	20.0%	0.71 (0.60–0.83)	< 0.01	48
LOWASA[27]	2002	3300	1.25 mg qd		75	27.1%	27.8%	np	ns	56

[a] *p*-value by Fisher exact test. [b] Mortality, primary end-point.
N, number of patients randomized; INR, international normalized ratio; ASA, aspirin; OAC, oral anticoagulation; 1° end-point, primary end-point; RR, relative risk; Fup, follow-up period; qd, 4 times a day; Good/Poor compliers: oral anticoagulation use in over/less than 70% patients at 35 days; ns, not significant; na, not applicable; np, not provided; mths, months; 95% CI, 95% confidence interval.
Unpublished data are shown as presented at the respective congresses, and are preliminary results. Modified from Brouwer and Verheugt (2002).[19]

a logical follow-up therapy following discontinuation of heparin in thrombotic disorders. The impact of oral anticoagulation is effected by interference with the production of vitamin K-dependent coagulation factors (II, VII, IX, X).[19]

As a single antithrombotic regimen after myocardial infarction (MI), it has been tested extensively during the past three decades.[19] Not until recently, however, has the combination of oral anticoagulation with the standard antiplatelet regimen after MI (aspirin) been evaluated. This combination has become more appealing since the introduction of lower doses of aspirin (maximum 325 mg daily), and the improved safety of oral anticoagulation following the introduction of the international normalized ratio (INR).

In the CARS trial, over 9000 patients, early after MI, were randomized to aspirin alone (daily dose 160 mg), or to aspirin (80 mg daily) combined with fixed-dose warfarin (1 or 3 mg daily) and reached INRs 1.1 and 1.5, respectively.[20] After 1.2 years no differences were observed in mortality and recurrent MI. Similar disappointing results were seen after 2.5 years in the over 5000 patients' CHAMP study, with a reached INR of 1.8. In that trial, patients were randomized to aspirin alone 160 mg daily or to aspirin 80 mg daily plus warfarin, which was laboratory-monitored to an INR of 1.5–2.5.[21]

Recently, two trials from the Netherlands on this topic have been carried out. The APRICOT-2 angiographic follow-up study investigated the role of combined anticoagulant (mean INR 2.6)/antiplatelet therapy versus aspirin alone (80 mg daily) in 308 patients with a patent infarct artery after fibrinolytic therapy.[22] To date, this is the only trial studying this combined antithrombotic regimen specifically in patients treated with fibrinolysis. The combined treatment reduced angiographic reocclusion at 3 months from 28% with aspirin to 15% ($p < 0.02$). Although secondary end-points, recurrent infarction and the need for revascularization were markedly reduced on the prolonged combined antithrombotic regimen and safety was excellent (no intracranial haemorrhage, only minor bleedings were doubled by Coumadin + aspirin). The clinical ASPECT-2 trial studied full intensity (mean INR 3.2) Coumadin alone (without aspirin), the combination Coumadin (mean INR 2.4) and aspirin 80 mg daily, and aspirin 80 mg daily alone in 993 patients randomized within 2 weeks after myocardial infarction.[23] About 50% of the patients had received fibrinolytic therapy in the acute phase. The 1 year death and reinfarction rate of 8% on aspirin alone was reduced by 45% and 50% in the combination and Coumadin alone groups, respectively ($p = 0.05$). Also in this trial, bleeding was extremely low (major bleeding for the combination 1.8%, for aspirin alone 0.9%). However, despite promising efficacy findings, both trials are too small to be conclusive on safety.

The WARIS-II trial has been carried out in Norway in 3600 patients, who survived MI, and compares aspirin (160 mg daily) alone with either full-intensity oral anticoagulation (target INR 2.8–4.2) alone or the combination of low-dose aspirin (75 mg daily) with medium-intensity oral anticoagulation (target INR 2.0–2.5). Over a 4 year follow-up period, a 30% reduction in the combined end-point of death, reinfarction and stroke was observed with medium-intensity warfarin (mean INR 2.2) plus aspirin as compared to aspirin alone.[24]

In contrast to the larger clinical trials, in APRICOT-2, Coumadin was initiated early, within 48 hours of fibrinolysis, during heparinization.[22] Parenteral anticoagulation was discontinued when the target INR was reached: thus, an uninterrupted, prolonged combined antithrombotic regimen was obtained. A similar strategy was followed in a smaller angiographic trial performed in a mixed patient population recovering from acute coronary syndromes and reported similar findings.[25] Clinically, this may offer additional benefit, as the majority of recurrent events occurs within the first 5–7 days. The only clinical trial with this regimen was OASIS-2, addressing non-ST-elevation acute coronary syndromes.[26] Importantly, a stratified comparison on the compliance per centre showed that the potential efficacy was largely dependent on the level of compliance (see Table 4.3).

The positive impact of Coumadin on long-term reocclusion and recurrent ischaemic events seems to corroborate well with the in-hospital clinical benefit seen with the new prolonged antithrombin regimens in the angiographic studies,[12–14] and the clinical ASSENT-3 trial.[16]

Recently, the Swedish LOWASA trial has been completed, which evaluated combined fixed low-dose oral anticoagulation (1.25 mg daily) and antiplatelet therapy (aspirin 75 mg daily) in comparison to aspirin alone (75 mg daily) in 3300 post-MI patients. The primary end-point was not affected, whereas severe bleeding was increased on the combined regimen. Data on the reached intensity of anticoagulation are awaited.[27]

Thus, adding oral anticoagulants to antiplatelet therapy does not improve outcome when the reached INR is below 2.0. Dose-adjusted, adequate anticoagulation with INRs over 2.0 seems to improve clinical and angiographic results after acute myocardial infarction.

Conclusions

Anticoagulants seem to be essential for improving outcome after fibrinolytic therapy for acute myocardial infarction. In the acute phase, unfractionated heparin (UFH) is widely used and does not seem to be inferior to direct thrombin inhibitors, such as hirudin and hirulog. Both LMWH and the specific Xa inhibitor pentasaccharide could be excellent, more practical alternatives. Although in-hospital reocclusion and recurrent ischaemic events seem lower with a regimen of an i.v. bolus of

LMWH followed by subcutaneous injections until discharge, its safety is still a matter of debate.

Following the acute phase, dose-adjusted Coumadin plus aspirin seems to provide additional benefit after myocardial infarction, when compared to aspirin alone. Important issues are timing and adequacy of the intensity of therapy. Anticoagulation with INRs below 2.0 does not translate into better outcomes following myocardial infarction. Bleeding is acceptable since the introduction of lower doses of aspirin, but more trials are necessary to confirm efficacy and safety.

In view of these findings, studies on Xa inhibitors that can be administered once weekly and the current trials with oral direct thrombin inhibitors might result in attractive alternatives for Coumadin, without the need of monitoring.

References

1. Fibrinolytics Therapy Trialists' Collaborative Group. Indications for fibrinolytic therapy in suspected acute myocardial infarction: collaborative overview of early mortality and major morbidity results from all randomised trials of more than 1000 patients. Lancet 1994; **343**:311–22.

2. Morrison LJ, Verbeek PR, McDonald AC, Sawadsky BV, Cook DJ. Mortality and pre-hospital thrombolysis for acute myocardial infarction: A meta-analysis. JAMA 2000; **283**:2686–92.

3. Collins R, Peto R, Baigent C, Sleight P. Aspirin, heparin, and fibrinolytic therapy in acute myocardial infarction. N Engl J Med 1997; **336**:847–60.

4. Verheugt FWA, Meijer A, Lagrand WK, Van Eenige MJ. Reocclusion, the flipside of coronary thrombolysis. J Am Coll Cardiol 1996; **27**:766–73.

5. Granger CB, Hirsh J, Califf RM et al. Activated partial thromboplastin time and outcome after thrombolytic therapy for acute myocardial infarction: results from the GUSTO-1 trial. Circulation 1996; **93**:870–8.

6. Gore JM, Granger CB, Sloan MA et al. Stroke after thrombolysis: mortality and functional outcome after thrombolytic therapy for acute myocardial infarction: results from the GUSTO trial. Circulation 1995; **92**:2811–18.

7. Gugliano RP, McCabe CH, Antman EM et al. Lower-dose heparin with fibrinolysis is associated with lower rates of intracranial hemorrhage. Am Heart J 2001; **141**:742–50.

8. Van de Werf F, Ardissino D, Betriu A et al. Management of acute myocardial infarction in patients presenting with ST-elevation. Eur Heart J 2003; **24**:28–66.

9. GUSTO-IIb investigators. A comparison of recombinant hirudin with heparin for the treatment of acute coronary syndromes. N Engl J Med 1996; **335**:775–82.

10. Antman EM for the TIMI-9B investigators. Hirudin in acute myocardial infarction. Thrombolysis In Myocardial Infarction (TIMI) 9B trial. Circulation 1994; **90**:1624–30.

11. HERO-2 investigators. Thrombin-specific anticoagulation with bivalirudin versus heparin in

patients receiving fibrinolytic therapy for acute myocardial infarction: the HERO-2 trial. Lancet 2001; **358**:1855–63.

12. Wallentin L, Dellborg DM, Lindahl B, Nilsson T, Pehrsson K, Swahn E. The low-molecular-weight heparin dalteparin as adjuvant therapy in acute myocardial infarction: the ASSENT PLUS study. Clin Cardiol 2001; **24**(suppl 1):12–14.

13. Ross AM, Molhoek P, Lundergan C et al. Randomized comparison of enoxaparin, a low molecular weight heparin, with unfractionated heparin adjunctive to tissue plasminogen activator thrombolysis and aspirin: second trial of Heparin and Aspirin Reperfusion Therapy (HART II). Circulation 2001; **104**:648–52.

14. Simoons ML, Alonso A, Krzeminska-Pakula M et al. Early ST segment elevation resolution: Predictor of outcome and angiographic patency in patients with acute myocardial infarction. Results of the AMI-SK study. Eur Heart J 2002; **23**:1282–90.

15. Coussement PK, Bassand JP, Convens C et al. A synthetic factor-Xa inhibitor (ORG13540/SR9017A) as an adjunct to fibrinolysis in acute myocardial infarction. The PENTALYSE-study. Eur Heart J 2001; **22**:1716–24.

16. ASSENT-3 investigators. Efficacy and safety of tenecteplase with enoxaparin, abciximab or unfractionated heparin: the ASSENT-3 randomised trial in acute myocardial infarction. Lancet 2001; **358**:605–13.

17. Wallentin L. One year follow-up data of the ASSENT-3 trial. Presented at the 24th Congress of the European Society of Cardiology, 31 August to 4 September 2002, Berlin, Germany.

18. Wallentin L. The ASSENT3-PLUS trial. Presented at the 75th Scientific Sessions of the American Heart Association, 17–20 November 2002, Chicago, IL, USA.

19. Brouwer MA, Verheugt FWA. Oral anticoagulants in acute coronary syndromes. Circulation 2002; **105**:1270–4.

20. Coumadin Aspirin Reinfarction Study (CARS) investigators. Randomised double-blind trial of fixed low-dose warfarin with aspirin after myocardial infarction. Lancet 1997; **350**:389–96.

21. Fiore LD, Ezekowitz MD, Brophy MT et al. for the Combination Hemotherapy and Mortality Prevention (CHAMP) Study Group. Department of Veteran Affairs cooperative studies program clinical trial comparing combined warfarin and aspirin with aspirin alone in survivors of acute myocardial infarction. Primary results of the CHAMP study. Circulation 2002; **105**:557–63.

22. Brouwer MA, Van den Bergh PJPC, Vromans RPJW et al. Aspirin plus coumarin versus aspirin alone in the prevention of reocclusion after fibrinolysis for acute myocardial infarction: results of the APRICOT-2 trial. Circulation 2002; **106**:659–65.

23. Van Es RF, Jonker JJC, Verheugt FWA, Deckers JW, Grobbee DE. Aspirin and coumadin after acute coronary syndromes (the ASPECT-2 study): a randomised controlled trial. Lancet 2002; **360**:109–13.

24. Hurlen M, Abdelnoor M, Smith P, Erikssen J, Arnesen H. Warfarin, aspirin, or both after myocardial infarction. N Engl J Med 2002; **347**:969–74.

25. Williams MJA, Morison IM, Parker JH, Stewart RH. Progression of the culprit lesion

in unstable coronary artery disease with warfarin and aspirin versus aspirin alone: preliminary study. J Am Coll Cardiol 1997; **30**:364–9.

26. The Organisation to Assess Strategies for Ischemic Syndromes (OASIS-2) investigators. Effects of long-term, moderate-intensity oral anticoagulation in addition to aspirin in unstable angina. J Am Coll Cardiol 2001; **37**:475–84.

27. Herlitz J. Effect of low dose warfarin added to aspirin long term after acute myocardial infarction on cardiovascular death, reinfarction and stroke. Circulation 2002; **106**(suppl II): 320 (Abstract).

5

Pharmacological interventions for acute myocardial infarction

Preet Randhawa and William D Weaver

Introduction

Acute ST-elevation myocardial infarction (AMI) is usually caused by the rupture of an atherosclerotic plaque with subsequent thrombosis of the coronary artery.[1] It is associated with a high risk of morbidity and mortality, which has improved considerably in the past few decades with the development of better monitoring and immediate defibrillation in cardiac intensive care units along with improved antiischaemic, cardioprotective and reperfusion therapies. Reperfusion of the occluded coronary artery with thrombolytic therapy has been shown to reduce infarct size and preserve left ventricular (LV) function but most importantly has an even larger effect on improving overall survival.[2,3] AMI, however, remains the leading cause of morbidity and mortality in the United States with 600 000 deaths annually. Patients surviving an AMI remain at a higher risk for reinfarction and sudden death.

After coronary occlusion there is a wavefront progression of myocardial necrosis. The necrosis proceeds from the subendocardium to the subepicardium.[5] Early reperfusion has the potential of salvaging ischaemic myocardium especially in the subepicardial region. Thrombolytic drug therapy, primary percutaneous transluminal coronary angioplasty (PTCA) and various adjunctive therapies are aimed at causing early restoration of flow, preventing reocclusion and reducing ischaemia and infarct size, which ultimately determines the prognosis in these patients.

The window of opportunity for reperfusion in which there is greatest benefit of reducing morbidity and mortality is short. Although effective for 12 hours, most of the mortality reduction associated with reperfusion therapy is in the first 3 hours of MI.[6] The delay in the administration of thrombolytic drugs is probably the most important factor determining the benefit from therapy. The goal of reperfusion therapy is to attain complete and sustained arterial patency, especially TIMI-3 or normal flow. In a meta-analysis of thrombolytic trials, mortality was significantly lower for TIMI-3 flow (3.7%) as compared to TIMI-2 (7%) and TIMI-0 or TIMI-11 (8.8%).[7]

Currently, even with the use of the best thrombolytic regimen, complete reperfusion is achieved in only half of the patients.[9] To date, no agent since tissue plasminogen activator (t-PA) has shown higher patency rates. Reteplase and tenecteplase have the advantage of bolus administration and tenecteplase may cause less bleeding. Streptokinase is still the most widely used agent on a global basis despite its limitations. It does not require heparin and therefore may also cause less bleeding in high-risk patients.

There is a significant risk after adequate reperfusion of either intermittent or persistent reocclusion. Even though thrombolytic agents result in a 20% reduction in all-cause mortality, recurrent coronary events may occur in up to 40% of the patients during follow-up for 6 months.[3] Reocclusion appears to occur in a third of patients,[4] and recurrent ischaemia may result in infarct extension and an increased risk of death or MI.[8]

Thrombolytic drug therapy is also associated with activation of platelets and the coagulation pathway,[10] and further activation may occur with reperfusion. The excess mortality in the first day after reperfusion with thrombolytic therapy may be related to reperfusion injury.[3] The use of adjuvant therapy may play a role in extending the short window of opportunity and in achieving and maintaining complete reperfusion and reducing reperfusion injury. The mainstay for early reperfusion in most institutions in the United States remains thrombolytic therapy due to the lack of widespread availability of primary PTCA facilities except in tertiary care hospitals.

Beta blockers

The benefits of beta blocker therapy in reducing morbidity and mortality in AMI were demonstrated in the early 1980s in the prethrombolytic era and subsequently confirmed by several large clinical trials with metoprolol, atenolol, propranolol, timolol, etc.[10,12]

The mechanisms of action of beta blockers are as follows:

1. Reduce ischaemia and chest pain by decreasing the oxygen requirements of the myocardium. Decreasing heart rate, myocardial contractility, wall stress and blood pressure accomplishes this antiischaemic effect.
2. Reduce infarct size.
3. Increase the ventricular fibrillation threshold, resulting in a lower incidence of ventricular fibrillation and sustained ventricular tachycardia that may occur during reperfusion.[16]
4. Reduce risk of cardiac rupture, especially in patients receiving thrombolytic therapy.
5. Long-term use appears to prevent both recurrent MI and unexpected cardiac arrest.

Both beta blocker and thrombolytic drug therapy have been demonstrated to reduce recurrent ischaemia in the setting of an AMI. There are also improved survival rates and a reduced rate of recurrent AMI after the index event. There have been no large-scale trials to show the mortality benefit of beta blocker therapy in patients getting thrombolytic drug therapy. Since the mechanism of action for beta blockers and thrombolytic drugs is different the beneficial effects are potentially additive.

In the prethrombolytic era, the First International Study of Infarct Survival (ISIS-1) enrolled 16 027 patients with suspected AMI.[72] Patients were randomized to intravenous (i.v.) atenolol (5–10 mg) and then 100 mg/day for 7 days versus controls. There was a 15% relative reduction in mortality in the first week, which persisted to 1 year. There were also fewer cardiac arrest and reinfarctions.[11] Similar results have been shown with early administration of metoprolol.[12] A meta-analysis of more than 27 000 with an AMI demonstrated that treatment with beta blockers was associated with a 13% overall reduction in mortality. Additionally, there was also a reduction in non-fatal reinfarction (19%) and cardiac arrest (16%).[13]

In the thrombolytic era, the Thrombolysis in Myocardial Infarction (TIMI) IIB trial randomized 2948 patients to early and late beta blocker therapy with metoprolol (5 mg i.v. × 3, 50 mg twice daily for day 1 and then 100 mg twice daily) and rt-PA. Early intravenous administration of beta blockers was shown to be safe in combination with thrombolytic drug therapy. However, early therapy did not reduce overall mortality (possibly related to insufficient statistical power) and no difference was seen in regional and global LV function or arrhythmias between the groups.[14] The early therapy group, however, had a lower risk of recurrent chest pain, reinfarction and there was also a reduction in mortality in the low-risk subgroup at 6 weeks.

There are several theoretical benefits of the combination of beta blocker and thrombolytic therapy.

1. There is a reduced risk of cardiac rupture in patients receiving beta blockers. The risk of cardiac rupture is increased with the use of thrombolytic therapy, especially when treatment is delayed after onset of symptoms.
2. Suppression of tachyarrhythmias, which are associated with reperfusion.
3. A potential decrease in the risk of cerebral haemorrhage was suggested from the results of a *post hoc* analysis. Patients treated with 100 mg of t-PA who received immediate beta blocker therapy had an incidence of intracranial haemorrhage of 0% compared with a 0.8% in those who received delayed therapy.[14]

A possible mechanism for the reduced risk of intracranial haemorrhage may be related to a decrease in cerebral blood flow by permitting unopposed alpha adrenoreceptor-mediated vasoconstriction. It may also be associated with a decrease in blood pressure; however, this possible protective effect was not seen with other antihypertensive agents.

Even with the compelling evidence of the benefits of beta blockers in patients with AMI they remain significantly underutilized and often are used at suboptimal doses.[14,15] Analysis of the records of approximately 200 000 patients with AMI shows only 34% of the patients received beta blockers. The percentage was even lower in the elderly, African-Americans and in patients with LV dysfunction, chronic obstructive pulmonary disease (COPD), insulin-dependent diabetes mellitus (IDDM), coronary heart failure (CHF) and elevated creatinine. There was a 40% reduction in mortality with beta blocker therapy. There was a somewhat lower percentage reduction in mortality in the higher-risk patients; however, since their absolute mortality was higher, the absolute reduction was significant.

Current recommendations for beta blocker in AMI is to use in all patients without a contraindication who can be treated within 12 hours of onset of symptoms, irrespective of the administration of concomitant thrombolytic therapy or performance of primary angioplasty and in patients with ongoing ischaemia and tachyarrhythmias. They should also be continued lifelong in all patients without contraindications.[17]

Contraindications to the use of beta blockers in AMI are asthma or active bronchospasm, hypotension, significant pulmonary oedema and severe or symptomatic bradycardia.

Angiotensin-converting enzyme (ACE) inhibitors

The use of ACE inhibitors has been extensively evaluated in patients with heart failure and has shown a reduction in morbidity and mortality.[18,20] Similar beneficial effects have been seen in patients with an AMI. Following acute necrosis, the LV may undergo remodelling and progressive dilatation, which may lead to formation of an aneurysm. This is associated with deterioration of systolic function and an increase in mortality.[19] Reduction of this infarct expansion and remodelling by ACE inhibitors results in improved LV function and improvement in clinical outcomes.[22,23]

As compared to the beneficial effects of oral ACE inhibitors, infusion of intravenous enalapril in the Cooperative New Scandinavian Enalapril Survival Study II (CONSENSUS-II) trial was associated with a higher incidence of early hypotension and a trend towards increase in mortality (not significant) which led to premature termination of the trial.[21]

The mechanisms of action of ACE inhibitors are as follows:

1. Reduce LV remodelling and post-infarct expansion, resulting in improved LV function.[22]
2. Reduce incidence of recurrent ischaemia and MI.[22]
3. Reduce cardiovascular and overall mortality, by 20%, including incidence of sudden death by decreasing recurrent ischaemia and infarct expansion.
4. Possible direct effects on the endothelium and plaque stabilization.

The Survival And Ventricular Enlargement (SAVE) trial enrolled 2231 patients with ejection fraction (EF) < 40% without active ischaemia or overt heart failure. Patients were randomized to either captopril or placebo 3–16 days post-MI. The treated patients had a relative reduction in mortality of 19%, incidence of recurrent myocardial infarctions by 25% and less progression to heart failure. These benefits were seen in patients receiving thrombolytic drug therapy, aspirin and beta blockers and patients not receiving these drugs.[22] Similarly, the use of ramipril in post-MI patients with heart failure was associated with a reduction in mortality by 27% and a decrease in risk of developing severe heart failure.[24]

In the large, Fourth International Study of Infarct Survival (ISIS-4) 58 050 patients with suspected AMI were randomized within 24 hours to oral captopril therapy versus placebo. There was a 7% relative reduction in mortality (7.19% vs 7.69%) in the captopril group at 5 weeks in this largely unselected group of patients. The use of antiplatelet and thrombolytic therapy was 94% and 70%, respectively.[74] The GISSI-3 study showed a similar early benefit using lisinopril (11%); however, at 6 months the difference in mortality was non-significant except in those patients at 'high risk' (anterior location, history of prior MI, etc.).[73] The use of thrombolytic drug therapy in these trials was high.[73,74] Benefits of ACE inhibitors, however, also extend to patients who do not receive thrombolytic therapy. In patients with acute anterior MI who did not receive reperfusion therapy use of ACE inhibitor zofenopril was associated with a reduction in mortality (25%) and development of severe coronary heart failure (CHF) at 6 weeks.[25]

Currently, therapy with ACE inhibitors within 24 hours is recommended in all patients with AMI (especially in the anterior location) and in patients with EF < 40% and CHF due to systolic dysfunction. Patients with symptomatic LV dysfunction or EF< 40% at 4–6 weeks post-MI should have ACE inhibitors continued long term. However, in patients with near normal LV function withdrawal of therapy may be considered.[17]

Calcium channel blockers

Calcium has been felt to have a prominent role in cellular injury during ischaemia and reperfusion. Various mechanisms have been postulated for the potential benefits of calcium channel blockers in myocardial ischaemia and reperfusion based on experimental data.

The mechanisms of action of calcium channel blockers are as follows:

1. Calcium channel antagonists reduce myocardial stunning and infarct size in MI with and without reperfusion.
2. They have antiplatelet effects, reduce neutrophil accumulation, reperfusion injury and the severity of microvascular damage in ischaemic tissue.

3. Rate-slowing calcium channel blockers reduce ischaemia by reducing myocardial oxygen demand and vasodilatation of epicardial vessels.
4. Calcium channel blockers preserve metabolism of high energy phosphates.

Despite the above theoretical benefits, a reduction in mortality has not been observed and, in fact, a number of trials have shown trends towards adverse outcome after treatment.[30,32] A meta-analysis of clinical trials of calcium channel blockers in the prethrombolytic era included 19 000 patients and showed a trend towards increased all-cause mortality (odds ratio 1.06; 95% CI 0.96–1.18). However, subgroup analysis showed that the heart rate slowing agents (verapamil and diltiazem) were different from vasodilators, which resulted in tachycardia and fewer reinfarctions were found in this group.[26]

Calcium channel blockers may be associated with an increased risk of bleeding which may be related to antiplatelet and vasodilatory properties. In the TIMI-II trial in which t-PA was used, the risk of intracerebral haemorrhage was four times higher in patients receiving calcium channel blockers at study entry versus those not on the drugs, although this has not been confirmed in other studies.[27] Similar results have been seen in patients undergoing cardiac surgery.[28]

Calcium channel antagonists are a diverse group with significantly different properties and can be divided into predominantly vasodilators (nifedipine) and heart rate slowing drugs (verapamil and diltiazem).

Nifedipine

Dihydropyridines, such as nifedipine, are vasodilators with a higher selectivity for vascular smooth muscle than the myocardium. This can lead to reflex tachycardia, especially with the use of short-acting preparations. Use of nifedipine, early or delayed therapy, after an AMI has not been shown to reduce risk of mortality or reinfarction.[29,75] Some trials have in fact shown a trend towards increased mortality.[75] A group of patients with AMI receiving thrombolytic therapy in combination with nifedipine showed no significant improvement in LV function, or mortality. The evolution of CK-MB (creatine kinase myoglobin fraction) release and cumulative CK-MB was higher in the treatment group as compared to the control group.[30] In another study, in post-MI patients both nifedipine and diltiazem showed a trend towards increase in adverse events.[31] A meta-analysis of 16 randomized trials demonstrated that the use of nifedipine was associated with an increase in relative risk of mortality to 1.16 (95% CI 1.01–1.33) and was dose-dependent.[32]

These adverse effects may be mediated by reflex tachycardia, 'coronary steal', hypotension, increased intracerebral haemorrhage (ICH), negative inotropic effects, etc.

Recommendations
Nifedipine (short-acting) is contraindicated in the treatment of AMI.[17]

Diltiazem

Diltiazem has been studied in AMI patients with and without thrombolytic drug therapy. In the prethrombolytic era, the Multicenter Diltiazem Post Infarction Trial (MDPIT) was a long-term trial of diltiazem prophylaxis in post-MI patients:[76] 2446 post-MI patients were randomized to diltiazem 240 mg/day or placebo, and were followed for a mean of 25 months. There was no difference in mortality within groups. There was an 11% reduction in first recurrent cardiac events (death from cardiac cause and non-fatal reinfarction), which was non-significant. However in subgroup analysis (which may not be statistically valid) of 80% post-MI patients without LV dysfunction, there was a significant reduction in cardiac events (cardiac death rate and non-fatal reinfarction). Of the patients with LV dysfunction (EF less than 40%) there was a significant increase in late cardiac event rates.[76] In another contemporary study in patients with non-Q-wave myocardial infarction (NQMI) there was approximately a 50% reduction in reinfarction and occurrence of refractory post infarction angina.[33]

William Boden and others have postulated that MI followed by thrombolysis may be similar to an NQMI. There is 'incomplete infarction' following successful reperfusion, preventing infarct expansion and development of aneurysm. Various similarities exist with NQMI, thus postulating a potential role for heart rate slowing calcium antagonist in patients with MI undergoing thrombolysis.[34] The Incomplete Infarction Trial of European Research Collaborators Evaluation Prognosis post-Thrombolysis (INTERCEPT) was designed to test this hypothesis. Patients without heart failure were randomized to diltiazem 36–96 hours post-thrombolysis. Diltiazem did not reduce the cumulative occurrence of cardiac death, non-fatal reinfarction, or refractory ischaemia during a 6 month follow-up. The composite of all end-points of non-fatal cardiac events were reduced, especially the need for revascularization.[35]

Other studies have reported improvement in LV function in patients with AMI treated with diltiazem and streptokinase.[36] The small DATA trial showed a reduction in mortality rate, reinfarction and recurrent ischaemia from 41% to 13% at 35 days and also reduced the need for urgent intervention. Most of the reduction was related to a reduction in recurrent ischaemia.[37]

Recommendations
In view of the above, diltiazem should not be used as a prophylactic agent in patients with reduced LV systolic function in the treatment of AMI.

Verapamil

Similar to diltiazem, verapamil was tested in the prethrombolytic era, in the Danish Verapamil Infarction Trial I (DAVIT I). Patients suspected of AMI were randomized early to verapamil or placebo. There was no overall benefit in the early phase and thereafter, on follow-up, there was a trend in favour of the verapamil group.[77] The late potentially beneficial effect of verapamil was further tested in the Danish Verapamil Infarction Trial II (DAVIT II), in which patients were randomized 7–15 days after a proven MI.[78] The use of verapamil in patients without heart failure showed a significant reduction in mortality (7.7% vs 11.8%) and rein-farction (9.4% vs 12.7%); however, there was no difference in mortality in patients with heart failure. The Calcium antagonist Reinfarction Italian Study (CRIS) in post-MI patients without CHF failed to show a benefit of verapamil on total mortality, cardiac death and sudden death.[40] There was a non-significant reduction in reinfarction rate and angina. The overall mortality in the CRIS trial was, however, lower than that in the DAVIT II due to the exclusion of higher-risk patients and may explain the difference.

The VISOR study evaluated LV function after acute anterior MI treated with early and prolonged administration of verapamil. All patients had been treated with thrombolysis. In those patients with EF of >45%, there was no improvement in systolic function but verapamil prevented alterations of diastolic function.[38] In a somewhat similar Verapamil in Acute Myocardial Infarction (VAMI) study there was a trend (statistically non-significant) towards lower end-diastolic and end-systolic volume at 90 days.[39]

Recommendations

Verapamil or diltiazem may be used in patients with contraindications to beta blockers with ongoing ischaemia, uncontrolled hypertension, or atrial fibrillation with rapid ventricular rate in the absence of coronary heart failure (CHF), LV dysfunction or heart block. Diltiazem may be used in patients with non-ST elevation MI without CHF or LV dysfunction.[17]

Magnesium

There have been several small trials that studied the role of magnesium in patients suspected to have an AMI and showed reduced mortality and a lower risk of ventricular arrhythmias. Subsequently, a meta-analysis of these trials showed significant benefits of magnesium therapy in reduc-ing mortality (by 55%) and the incidence of ventricular arrhythmias; it also had a significant beneficial effect on infarct size and left ventricular function.[41]

The mechanisms of action of magnesium are as follows:

1. Magnesium is an important cofactor in many enzymatic reactions and the concentration of magnesium is reduced after an AMI. At the same time, there is an increased requirement of magnesium to maintain metabolic processes.
2. In experimental models, magnesium protects against effects of oxygen free radicals, inhibits calcium overload of cells and reduces reperfusion injury.[42]
3. Magnesium is a potent vasodilator and may increase coronary perfusion by causing afterload reduction.[43]
4. There is a reduction of the risk of cardiac arrhythmias by the membrane stabilizing effects and conservation of intracellular adenosine 5'-triphosphate (ATP).[44]

Pretreatment with intravenous magnesium prior to reperfusion has been shown to reduce infarct size in experimental models.[45] It is also known from animal models that the timing of infusion is critical to its effects. Infusion of magnesium at the time of reperfusion resulted in a decrease in infarct size by half. However, when the infusion was delayed there was no infarct-limiting effect.[46]

These findings led to the investigation of magnesium therapy in the second Leicester Intravenous Magnesium Intervention Trial (LIMIT-2). Magnesium infusions were started at the same time as thrombolytic therapy and continued for 24 hours. It showed a 24% reduction in the 28 day mortality, and long-term follow-up showed a 16% reduction in all-cause mortality.[47] These results were not substantiated in the much larger ISIS-4 trial, which showed a trend towards increased mortality following treatment with magnesium, nor in the recently presented but not published trial Magnesium in Coronaries (MAGIC). A criticism of the ISIS-4 trial was the significant delay between thrombolysis and the magnesium infusion. Reperfusion may already have occurred at the time of magnesium infusion, thus eliminating the chance for an effect.[74] The infusion of magnesium was also delayed from the onset of chest pain and adequate levels may not have been present in patients at the time of reperfusion. Magnesium therapy has also shown benefits in patients who were not candidates for reperfusion therapy.[48]

Recommendations
To date, there is insufficient evidence to support the routine use of magnesium in AMI. Current American College of Cardiology/American Heart Association (ACC/AHA) recommendations for magnesium therapy include correction of documented magnesium deficits and for episodes of torsades de pointes. Treatment for patients who are high risk, elderly or not candidates for thrombolytic therapy remains a TIMI-IIB recommendation.[17] In fact, the use of magnesium has for the most part stopped pending further study.

Nitrates

T Lauder Brunton first showed the antianginal effects of nitroglycerine in 1846. Several small clinical trials have shown benefits of nitrate therapy in AMI patients. The individual trials were, however, too small to show a mortality benefit. A meta-analysis of 10 trials by S Yusuf showed that the use of nitroglycerine or nitroprusside was associated with a 35% decrease in mortality.[49] The reduction was also non-significantly higher for nitroglycerine as compared to nitroprusside.

The mechanisms of action of nitrates are as follows:

1. Nitrates cause epicardial arterial and arteriolar dilatation with increase in perfusion to the ischaemic zone. They have been shown to cause more prompt reperfusion and an earlier improvement of LV function than reperfusion alone.[50]
2. Decrease in oxygen requirements by a decrease in preload, LV filling pressures and afterload. This results in a decrease in chest pain, myocardial ischaemia and ST elevation.
3. Reduce infarct size in experimental models along with an increase in collateral blood flow.[51]
4. Nitrates also have antiplatelet effects and can reduce the remodelling of the ventricle.

Given the potential benefits and findings of the meta-analysis the efficacy of nitrates was tested in two large randomized trials, GISSI-3 and ISIS-4. The GISSI-3 trial enrolled 18 895 patients to test efficacy of lisinopril and transdermal glyceryl trinitrate in patients with AMI. Patients were treated with other standard therapies including thrombolytics (72%), beta blockers (31%) and aspirin (84%). There was no reduction in mortality associated with nitrate therapy in this trial. However, a criticism of the GISSI-3 trial is that the non-protocol use of nitrates was more than 50%.[73] Similarly the ISIS-4 trial failed to demonstrate benefit for nitrate therapy.[74] However, a fewer number of deaths were seen between day 0 and 1. Like GISSI-3 the non-protocol use of nitrates was more than 50%. Given the large crossover rate, it is difficult to conclude anything except that the drugs are safe in this setting.

Recommendations

Routine use of nitrates in all patients with AMI is not recommended. They should be used in patients with recurrent ischaemia, coronary heart failure (CHF) or hypertension initially intravenously and then continued orally as required for symptom control.[17]

Lipid lowering drugs

Lipid lowering with HMGCoA reductase inhibitors (statins) has been shown in many trials to reduce death and ischaemic cardiovascular events.[52,53,57] These trials have also shown that lipid lowering can retard the progression of atherosclerosis throughout the vascular system and the benefits are maintained long term.[52]

Statins have also been shown to be effective in primary prevention of cardiovascular events,[54] and to reduce incidence of a transient ischaemic attack (TIA) and stroke.[53,54,55] However, most of these studies excluded patients with recent unstable angina or AMI and there is a high rate of death or recurrent ischaemic events in this population. There are several theoretical benefits for the use of lipid lowering therapy in this patient population:

1. Improved endothelial function.
2. Decrease in platelet aggregability and thrombus formation.
3. Stabilization of the unstable plaque with a decrease in low-density lipoprotein (LDL).

There is a growing move to use these agents immediately after acute coronary syndrome (ACS) or AMI; however, no trial has looked at benefits of immediate therapy in patients with acute ST-elevation MI with or without thrombolytic therapy. The results of the recent Myocardial Ischemia Reduction with Aggressive Cholesterol Lowering (MIRACL) trial showed that atorvastatin therapy in patients with ACS reduced recurrent ischaemic events; however, there was no reduction in death, MI or cardiac arrest.[56] The potential benefits of immediate treatment in patients with ST-elevation MI are unknown at this time.

Recommendations
ACC/AHA recommendations for AMI are diet therapy in all patients after MI and treatment for those with persistently elevated LDL to a target goal of less than 100 mg/dl.[17] In our own practice, we believe that hos-pitalization for ACS provides an opportunity to provide education and either initiate or optimize statin therapy. If the LDL is elevated in the first 24 hours, we begin treatment using a moderately high dose, which can be titrated down if needed in 4–6 weeks. This approach helps to ensure that more patients would be at target during the year following hospitalization as many are inadequately monitored after discharge from hospital.

Adenosine

Adenosine has been extensively studied in animal models as a cardio-protective agent and also in small clinical trials in humans to reduce reperfusion injury.

The mechanisms of action of adenosine:

1. Adenosine inhibits oxygen free radical formation and neutrophil activity.
2. Improvement of endothelial and microvascular function.

3. Improvement of collateral flow and participation in ischaemic preconditioning.

Adenosine has been studied in the Acute Myocardial Infarction STudy of ADenosine (AMISTAD) trial in patients receiving thrombolytic therapy.[57] Infusion of adenosine and lidocaine were used in patients presenting within 6 hours of onset of chest pain and showed a significant reduction in infarct size measured by single photon emission computed tomography (SPECT) imaging at an average of 6 days post-MI. There was a reduction in the infarct size of 67% in patients with anterior MI; however, no reduction was seen with other infarct locations. There was also a trend towards increased adverse events in the non-anterior sub-group. No additional benefit to the use of lidocaine in patients receiving adenosine infusions was seen and there was also no significant difference in clinical outcomes between treatment groups; however, the overall number of events was small. Similarly, in patients undergoing primary PTCA for AMI, intracoronary adenosine has been used and is associated with a higher rate of TIMI flow and lower incidence of no reflow.[58]

A larger trial has recently been completed, and failed to show a benefit of adenosine in patients treated with reperfusion therapy.

Glucose–insulin–potassium (GIK)

The concept of metabolic protection of ischaemic myocardium is based on the fact that glucose can be metabolized anaerobically by the glycolytic pathway and lead to the generation of ATP.[62] Insulin is added to the regimen to promote the entry of glucose into the cells and also facilitates cellular uptake of potassium. A meta-analysis of nine trials with about 1900 patients showed a 28% reduction in in-hospital mortality.[60]

The Latin American randomized ECLA trial used both low- and high-dose GIK infusions. There was a reduction in adverse cardiac events in the treatment group and this reached statistical significance in patients who underwent reperfusion therapy, which was mostly accomplished with thrombolytic therapy. The benefit was also greater for the high-dose GIK infusion.[61] However, in the Polish GIK trial, use of low-dose GIK infusion did not result in a difference in cardiac mortality and cardiac events between groups at 35 days. The overall mortality in the GIK group was significantly higher.[59] The major differences between the trials was a higher risk of mortality in the ECLA trial and the higher dose of GIK infusion.

Even though this therapy is easy to use and does not require expensive technology the efficacy is still uncertain. The results of ongoing larger trials are awaited before recommendations can be made regarding the routine use of GIK therapy.

Improvement of microvascular function

Optimal reperfusion has been redefined to include intact microvascular function and myocardial tissue perfusion in addition to complete and sustained epicardial artery patency. In addition to myocardial injury with ischaemia there is also injury to the coronary microvasculature and this may be further aggravated by reperfusion. The open artery hypothesis suggests that sustained patency of the epicardial artery results in improvement of LV function and a reduction in adverse clinical events. However, approximately 25% of the patients with TIMI-3 flow in the epicardial artery after AMI do not have adequate myocardial tissue reperfusion and it is an independent predictor of poor recovery of LV function.[63]

Even though reperfusion of ischaemic myocardium can reduce infarct size and mortality in patients with AMI, there is evidence that reperfusion can cause further injury to ischaemic cells. Reperfusion may lead to myocardial stunning, arrhythmias and even lethal cellular injury. The actual mechanism of reperfusion injury and microvascular dysfunction has not been elucidated. The aetiology is believed to be multifactorial and inhibition of several potential mechanisms of reperfusion injury has been attempted with drug therapy.

Platelets

Thrombolysis does not affect the platelet component of the thrombus and platelet micro-emboli generated from the lysis of the thrombus can lead to obstruction of the microvasculature. In addition, thrombolytic drug therapy can cause an increased production of thrombin and result in further platelet activation. Products from activated platelets may lead to spasm of the microvasculature, resulting in slow flow or no reflow.

Platelet glycoprotein (GP) IIb/IIIa inhibitors have been used as adjunctive therapy for both thrombolytic therapy and primary PTCA and have shown promising results.[64] They appear to accelerate the resolution of ST segments, a marker of myocardial reperfusion. Additionally, aspirin is indicated in all patients with an AMI or coronary arterial disease (CAD) and the use of clopidogrel is increasing in this patient population.

Neutrophils

Neutrophil activation and plugging occurs with reperfusion of the ischaemic myocardium. This results in neutrophil accumulation in the myocardium and has been associated with no reflow in experimental studies. Depletion of neutrophils,[65] or inhibition of neutrophil adhesion,[66] reduces endothelial dysfunction. Two phase II studies testing an anti-CD 11,18,[80] and CD 18 antibodies,[79] in the setting of thrombolysis and primary PTCA, failed to show a reduction in infarct size following treatment. The studies were not large enough to assess clinical events.

Complement inhibition

Complement activation occurs in AMI and deposition of complement components has been shown in the ischaemic myocardium.[67] Activation of complement results in chemotaxis and activation of neutrophils, resulting in infiltration of the ischaemic myocardium by neutrophils. This leads to tissue inflammation and also the release of oxygen free radicals. Increased levels of C5b-9, an important mediator of ischaemic tissue injury, have been seen in patients with AMI. Depletion or inhibition of complement has been shown to reduce reperfusion injury in experimental models. Anti-C5 therapy resulted in significant inhibition of cell apoptosis, necrosis and neutrophil accumulation in an experimental model.[68] Use of complement inhibition in addition to thrombolytic or PTCA therapy is being tested in the COMPLY and COMMA trials, respectively.

Oxygen free radicals

Oxygen free radicals are generated during reperfusion of ischaemic tissue and there is experimental evidence that suggests they play an important role in reperfusion injury. There is conflicting evidence of the efficacy of anti-free radical therapies on myocardial infarct size. Use of superoxide dismutase (SOD) as an adjunctive therapy to thrombolysis failed to show benefits in patients with AMI.[69] A similar trial in patients with anterior MI undergoing PTCA failed to demonstrate a beneficial effect of SOD on global or regional LV function.[70] Similarly, the effects of fluosol, an oxygen-carrying fluorocarbon were initially promising; however, the results of subsequent larger trials were disappointing.[71]

Calcium

Disturbances in calcium homeostasis also play a role in the pathogenesis of reperfusion injury and the use of calcium channel antagonist may attenuate reperfusion injury.

Various therapies are being tested in an effort to reduce reperfusion injury and improve microvascular function and have the potential, in the future, of further improving the efficacy of thrombolytic therapy. However, to date, none have shown any benefit.

References

1. DeWood MA, Spores J, Notske R, Mouser LT, Burroughs R, Golden MS, Lang HT. Prevalence of total coronary occlusion during the early hours of transmural myocardial infarction. N Engl J Med 1980; **303**:897–902.

2. GISSI investigators. Effectiveness of intravenous thrombolytic

treatment in acute myocardial infarction. Gruppo Italiano per lo Studio della Streptochinasi nell'Infarto Miocardico (GISSI). Lancet 1986; **1**:397–402.

3. FTT investigators. Indications for fibrinolytic therapy in suspected acute myocardial infarction: collaborative overview of early mortality and major morbidity results from all randomised trials of more than 1000 patients. Fibrinolytic Therapy Trialists' (FTT) Collaborative Group. Lancet 1994; **343**:311–22.

4. Meijer A, Verheugt FW, Werter CJ, Lie KI, van der Pol JM, van Eenige MJ. Aspirin versus coumadin in the prevention of reocclusion and recurrent ischemia after successful thrombolysis: a prospective placebo-controlled angiographic study. Results of the APRICOT Study. Circulation 1993; **87**:1524–30.

5. Reimer KA, Jennings RB. The "wavefront phenomenon" of myocardial ischemic cell death: II. Transmural progression of necrosis within the framework of ischemic bed size (myocardium at risk) and collateral flow. Lab Invest 1979; **40**:633–44.

6. Gersh BJ, Anderson JL. Thrombolysis and myocardial salvage. Results of clinical trials and the animal paradigm—paradoxic or predictable? Circulation 1993; **88**:296–306.

7. Anderson JL, Karagounis LA, Califf RM. Metaanalysis of five reported studies on the relation of early coronary patency grades with mortality and outcomes after acute myocardial infarction. Am J Cardiol 1996; **78**:1–8.

8. Stone GW, Grines CL, Browne KF, Marco J, Rothbaum D, O'Keefe J, Hartzler GO, Overlie P, Donohue B, Chelliah N. Implications of recurrent ischemia after reperfusion therapy in acute myocardial infarction: a comparison of thrombolytic therapy and primary angioplasty. J Am Coll Cardiol 1995; **26**:66–72.

9. The GUSTO Angiographic investigators. The effects of tissue plasminogen activator, streptokinase, or both on coronary-artery patency, ventricular function, and survival after acute myocardial infarction. N Engl J Med 1993; **329**:1615–22.

10. Fitzgerald DJ, Wright F, FitzGerald GA. Increased thromboxane biosynthesis during coronary thrombolysis. Evidence that platelet activation and thromboxane A2 modulate the response to tissue-type plasminogen activator in vivo. Circulation Res 1989; **65**:83–94.

11. ISIS-1 investigators. Randomised trial of intravenous atenolol among 16 027 cases of suspected acute myocardial infarction: ISIS-1. First International Study of Infarct Survival Collaborative Group. Lancet 1986; **2**:57–66.

12. The MIAMI Trial Research Group. Metoprolol in Acute Myocardial Infarction (MIAMI). A randomized placebo-controlled international trial. Eur Heart J 1985; **6**:199.

13. Yusuf S, Sleight P, Held P, McMahon S. Routine medical management of acute myocardial infarction. Lessons from overviews of recent randomized controlled trials. Circulation 1990; **82**(suppl 3):II117–34.

14. Roberts R, Rogers WJ, Mueller HS, Lambrew CT, Diver DJ, Smith HC, Willerson JT, Knatterud GL, Forman S, Passamani E. Immediate versus deferred beta-blockade following thrombolytic therapy in patients with acute myocardial infarction. Results of the Thrombolysis in Myocardial Infarction (TIMI) II-B

Study. Circulation 1991; **83**: 422–37.

15. Gottlieb SS, McCarter RJ, Vogel RA. Effect of beta-blockade on mortality among high-risk and low-risk patients after myocardial infarction. N Engl J Med 1998; **339**:489–97.

16. Ryden L, Ariniego R, Arnman K, Herlitz J, Hjalmarson A, Holmberg S, Reyes C, Smedgard P, Svedberg K, Vedin A, Waagstein F, Waldenstrom A, Wilhelmsson C, Wedel H, Yamamoto M. A double-blind trial of metoprolol in acute myocardial infarction. Effects on ventricular tachyarrhythmias. N Engl J Med 1983; **308**:614–18.

17. Ryan TJ, Antman EM, Brooks NH, Califf RM, Hillis LD, Hiratzka LF, Rapaport E, Riegel B, Russell RO, Smith EE 3rd, Weaver WD, Gibbons RJ, Alpert JS, Eagle KA, Gardner TJ, Garson A Jr, Gregoratos G, Ryan TJ, Smith SC Jr. 1999 update: ACC/AHA guidelines for the management of patients with acute myocardial infarction. A report of the American College of Cardiology/American Heart Association Task Force on Practice Guidelines (Committee on Management of Acute Myocardial Infarction). J Am Coll Cardiol 1999; **34**: 890–911.

18. SOLVD investigators. Effect of enalapril on survival in patients with reduced left ventricular ejection fractions and congestive heart failure. The SOLVD investigators. N Engl J Med 1991; **325**:293–302.

19. Jeremy RW, Allman KC, Bautovitch G, Harris PJ. Patterns of left ventricular dilation during the six months after myocardial infarction. J Am Coll Cardiol 1989; **13**:304–10.

20. Cohn JN, Johnson G, Ziesche S, Cobb F, Francis G, Tristani F, Smith R, Dunkman WB, Loeb H, Wong M. A comparison of enalapril with hydralazine-isosorbide dinitrate in the treatment of chronic congestive heart failure. N Engl J Med 1991; **325**:303–10.

21. Swedberg K, Held P, Kjekshus J, Rasmussen K, Ryden L, Wedel H. Effects of the early administration of enalapril on mortality in patients with acute myocardial infarction. Results of the Co-operative New Scandinavian Enalapril Survival Study II (CONSENSUS II). N Engl J Med 1992; **327**:678–84.

22. Pfeffer MA, Braunwald E, Moye LA, Basta L, Brown EJ Jr, Cuddy TE, Davis BR, Geltman EM, Goldman S, Flaker GC. Effect of captopril on mortality and morbidity in patients with left ventricular dysfunction after myocardial infarction. Results of the survival and ventricular enlargement trial. The SAVE investigators. N Engl J Med 1992; **327**:669–77.

23. Vannam M, Taylor D, Esakoff D, Webb-Peploe M. Early enalapril therapy attenuates acute infarct expansion and late global ventricular dilatation after first myocardial infarction. Circulation 1993; **88**:I–395.

24. AIRE investigators. Effect of ramipril on mortality and morbidity of survivors of acute myocardial infarction with clinical evidence of heart failure. The Acute Infarction Ramipril Efficacy (AIRE) study investigators. Lancet 1993; **342**:821–8.

25. Ambrosioni E, Borghi C, Magnani B. The effect of the angiotensin-converting-enzyme inhibitor zofenopril on mortality and morbidity after anterior myocardial infarction. The Survival of Myocardial Infarction Long-Term Evaluation (SMILE) Study

Investigators. N Engl J Med 1995; **332**:80–5.

26. Held PH, Yusuf S, Furberg CD. Calcium channel blockers in acute myocardial infarction and unstable angina: an overview. BMJ 1989; **299**:1187–92.

27. Gore JM, Sloan M, Price TR, Randall AM, Bovill E, Collen D, Forman S, Knatterud GL, Sopko G, Terrin ML. Intracerebral hemorrhage, cerebral infarction, and subdural hematoma after acute myocardial infarction and thrombolytic therapy in the Thrombolysis in Myocardial Infarction Study. Thrombolysis in Myocardial Infarction: Phase II. pilot and clinical trial. Circulation 1991; **83**:448–59.

28. Wagenknecht LE, Furberg CD, Hammon JW, Legault C, Troost BT. Surgical bleeding: unexpected effect of a calcium antagonist. BMJ 1995; **310**:776–7.

29. Wilcox RG, Hampton JR, Banks DC, Birkhead JS, Brooksby IA, Burns-Cox CJ, Hayes MJ, Joy MD, Malcolm AD, Mather HG. Trial of early nifedipine in acute myocardial infarction: the Trent study. BMJ Clin Res edn 1986; **293**:1204–8.

30. Erbel R, Pop T, Meinertz T, Olshausen KV, Treese N, Henrichs KJ, Schuster CJ, Rupprecht HJ, Schlurmann W, Meyer J. Combination of calcium channel blocker and thrombolytic therapy in acute myocardial infarction. Am Heart J 1988; **115**:529–38.

31. Ishikawa K, Nakai S, Takenaka T, Kanamasa K, Hama J, Ogawa I, Yamamoto T, Oyaizu M, Kimura A, Yamamoto K, Yabushita H, Katori R. Short-acting nifedipine and diltiazem do not reduce the incidence of cardiac events in patients with healed myocardial infarction. Secondary Prevention Group. Circulation 1997; **95**:2368–73.

32. Furberg CD, Psaty BM, Meyer JV. Nifedipine. Dose-related increase in mortality in patients with coronary heart disease. Circulation 1995; **92**:1326–31.

33. Gibson RS, Boden WE, Theroux P, Strauss HD, Pratt CM, Gheorghiade M, Capone RJ, Crawford MH, Schlant RC, Kleiger RE. Diltiazem and reinfarction in patients with non-Q-wave myocardial infarction. Results of a double-blind, randomized, multicenter trial. N Engl J Med 1986; **315**:423–9.

34. Boden WE. Calcium-channel blockers as adjuvant therapy postthrombolysis. J Cardiovasc Pharmacol 1991; **18**(suppl 10):S102–6.

35. Boden WE, van Gilst WH, Scheldewaert RG, Starkey IR, Carlier MF, Julian DG, Whitehead A, Bertrand ME, Col JJ, Pedersen OL, Lie KI, Santoni JP, Fox KM. Diltiazem in acute myocardial infarction treated with thrombolytic agents: a randomised placebo-controlled trial. Incomplete Infarction Trial of European Research Collaborators Evaluating Prognosis post-Thrombolysis (INTERCEPT). Lancet 2000; **355**:1751–6.

36. Nicolau JC, Ramires JA, Maggioni AP, Garzon SA, Pinto MA, Silva DG, Nogueira PR, Maia LF, Vendramini P, Bassi I. Diltiazem improves left ventricular systolic function following acute myocardial infarction treated with streptokinase. The Calcium Antagonist in Reperfusion Study (CARES) Group. Am J Cardiol 1996; **78**:1049–52.

37. Theroux P, Gregoire J, Chin C, Pelletier G, de Guise P, Juneau M. Intravenous diltiazem in acute myocardial infarction. Diltiazem as Adjunctive Therapy to Activase (DATA) trial. J Am Coll Cardiol 1998; **32**:620–8.

38. Natale E, Tubaro M, Di Marcotullio G, Celli P, Carelli M, Malinconico U, Polizzi CA, Milazzotto F, Vajola SF. The effect of verapamil on left ventricular remodelling and diastolic function after acute myocardial infarction (the Verapamil Infarction Study on Remodelling and Relaxation—VISOR). Cardiovasc Drugs Ther 1999; **13**:315–24.

39. Marangelli V, Memmola C, Brigiani MS, Boni L, Biasco MG, Scrutinio D, Iliceto S, Rizzon P. Early administration of verapamil after thrombolysis in acute anterior myocardial infarction. Effect on left ventricular remodeling and clinical outcome. VAMI Study Group. Verapamil Acute Myocardial Infarction. Ital Heart J 2000; **1**:336–43.

40. Rengo F, Carbonin P, Pahor M, DeCaprio L, Bernabei R, Ferrara N, Carosella L, Acanfora D, Parlati S, Vitale D. A controlled trial of verapamil in patients after acute myocardial infarction: results of the Calcium antagonist Reinfarction Italian Study (CRIS). Am J Cardiol 1996; **77**:365–9.

41. Teo KK, Yusuf S, Collins R, Held PH, Peto R. Effects of intravenous magnesium in suspected acute myocardial infarction: overview of randomised trials. BMJ 1991; **303**:1499–503.

42. Atar D, Serebruany V, Poulton J, Godard J, Schneider A, Herzog WR. Effects of magnesium supplementation in a porcine model of myocardial ischemia and reperfusion. J Cardiovasc Pharmacol 1994; **24**:603–11.

43. Woods KL. Possible pharmacological actions of magnesium in acute myocardial infarction. Br J Clin Pharmacol 1991; **32**:3–10.

44. Roden DM. Magnesium treatment of ventricular arrhythmias. Am J Cardiol 1989; **63**:43G–46G.

45. Leor J, Kloner RA. An experimental model examining the role of magnesium in the therapy of acute myocardial infarction. Am J Cardiol 1995; **75**:1292–3.

46. Herzog WR, Schlossberg ML, MacMurdy KS, Edenbaum LR, Gerber MJ, Vogel RA, Serebruany VL. Timing of magnesium therapy affects experimental infarct size. Circulation 1995; **92**:2622–6.

47. Woods KL, Fletcher S, Roffe C, Haider Y. Intravenous magnesium sulphate in suspected acute myocardial infarction: results of the second Leicester Intravenous Magnesium Intervention Trial (LIMIT-2). Lancet 1992; **339**:1553–8.

48. Shechter M, Hod H, Chouraqui P, Kaplinsky E, Rabinowitz B. Magnesium therapy in acute myocardial infarction when patients are not candidates for thrombolytic therapy. Am J Cardiol 1995; **75**:321–3.

49. Yusuf S, Collins R, MacMahon S, Peto R. Effect of intravenous nitrates on mortality in acute myocardial infarction: an overview of the randomised trials. Lancet 1988; **1**:1088–92.

50. Jugdutt BI, Michorowski BL, Tymchak WJ. Improved left ventricular function and topography by prolonged nitroglycerin therapy after acute myocardial infarction. Zeitschrift Kardiol 1989; **78**(suppl 2):127–9 (Discussion 142–4).

51. Jugdutt BI, Becker LC, Hutchins GM, Bulkley BH, Reid PR, Kallman CH. Effect of intravenous nitroglycerin on collateral blood flow and infarct size in the conscious dog. Circulation 1981; **63**:17–28.

52. 4S investigators. Randomised trial of cholesterol lowering in 4444 patients with coronary heart

disease: the Scandinavian Simvastatin Survival Study (4S). Lancet 1994; **344**:1383–9.

53. LIPID investigators. The Long-term Intervention with Pravastatin in Ischemic Disease (LIPID) Study Group. N Engl J Med 1998; **339**:1349–57.

54. Gottleib SS, McCarter RJ, Vogel, RA. Influence of pravastatin and plasma lipids on clinical events in the West of Scotland Coronary Prevention Study (WOSCOPS). Circulation 1998; **97**:1440–5.

55. Plehn JF, Davis BR, Sacks FM, Rouleau JL, Pfeffer MA, Bernstein V, Cuddy TE, Moye LA, Piller LB, Rutherford J, Simpson LM, Braunwald E. Reduction of stroke incidence after myocardial infarction with pravastatin: the Cholesterol and Recurrent Events (CARE) study. The Care Investigators. Circulation 1999; **99**:216–23.

56. Schwartz GG, Olsson AG, Ezekowitz MD, Ganz P, Oliver MF, Waters D, Zeiher A, Chaitman BR, Leslie S, Stern T. Myocardial Ischemia Reduction with Aggressive Cholesterol Lowering (MIRACL) Study Investigators. Effects of atorvastatin on early recurrent ischemic events in acute coronary syndromes: the MIRACL study: a randomized controlled trial. JAMA 2001; **285**:1711–18.

57. Mahaffey KW, Puma JA, Barbagelata NA, DiCarli MF, Leesar MA, Browne KF, Eisenberg PR, Bolli R, Casas AC, Molina-Viamonte V, Orlandi C, Blevins R, Gibbons RJ, Califf RM, Granger CB. Adenosine as an adjunct to thrombolytic therapy for acute myocardial infarction: results of a multicenter, randomized, placebo-controlled trial: the Acute Myocardial Infarction STudy of ADenosine (AMISTAD)

trial. J Am Coll Cardiol 1999; **34**:1711–20.

58. Marzilli M, Orsini E, Marraccini P, Testa R. Beneficial effects of intracoronary adenosine as an adjunct to primary angioplasty in acute myocardial infarction. Circulation 2000; **101**:2154–9.

59. Ceremuzynski L, Budaj A, Czepiel A, Burzykowski T, Achremczyk P, Smielak-Korombel W, Maciejewicz J, Dziubinska J, Nartowicz E, Kawka-Urbanek T, Piotrowski W, Hanzlik J, CieSlinski A, Kawecka-Jaszcz K, Gessek J, Wrabec K. Low-dose glucose-insulin-potassium is ineffective in acute myocardial infarction: results of a randomized multicenter Pol-GIK trial. Cardiovasc Drugs Ther 1999; **13**:191–200.

60. Fath-Ordoubadi F, Beatt KJ. Glucose-insulin-potassium therapy for treatment of acute myocardial infarction: an overview of randomized placebo-controlled trials. Circulation 1997; **96**:1152–6.

61. Diaz R, Paolasso EA, Piegas LS, Tajer CD, Moreno MG, Corvalan R, Isea JE, Romero G. Metabolic modulation of acute myocardial infarction. The ECLA (Estudios Cardiologicos Latinoamerica) Collaborative Group. Circulation 1998; **98**:2227–34.

62. Opie LH. Glucose and the metabolism of ischaemic myocardium. Lancet 1995; **345**:1520–1.

63. Ito H, Tomooka T, Sakai N, Yu H, Higashino Y, Fujii K, Masuyama T, Kitabatake A, Minamino T. Lack of myocardial perfusion immediately after successful thrombolysis. A predictor of poor recovery of left ventricular function in anterior myocardial infarction. Circulation 1992; **85**:1699–705.

64. Antman EM, Giugliano RP, Gibson CM, McCabe CH,

Coussement P, Kleiman NS, Vahanian A, Adgey AA, Menown I, Rupprecht HJ, Van der Wieken R, Ducas J, Scherer J, Anderson K, Van de Werf F, Braunwald E. Abciximab facilitates the rate and extent of thrombolysis: results of the thrombolysis in myocardial infarction (TIMI) 14 trial. The TIMI 14 Investigators. Circulation 1999; **99**:2720–32.

65. Sheridan FM, Dauber IM, McMurtry IF, Lesnefsky EJ, Horwitz LD. Role of leukocytes in coronary vascular endothelial injury due to ischemia and reperfusion. Circulation Res 1991; **69**:1566–74.

66. Ma XL, Lefer DJ, Lefer AM, Rothlein R. Coronary endothelial and cardiac protective effects of a monoclonal antibody to intercellular adhesion molecule-1 in myocardial ischemia and reperfusion. Circulation 1992; **86**:937–46.

67. Pinckard RN, O'Rourke RA, Crawford MH, Grover FS, McManus LM, Ghidoni JJ, Storrs SB, Olson MS. Complement localization and mediation of ischemic injury in baboon myocardium. J Clin Invest 1980; **66**:1050–6.

68. Vakeva AP, Agah A, Rollins SA, Matis LA, Li L, Stahl GL. Myocardial infarction and apoptosis after myocardial ischemia and reperfusion: role of the terminal complement components and inhibition by anti-C5 therapy. Circulation 1998; **97**:2259–67.

69. Murohara Y, Yui Y, Hattori R, Kawai C. Effects of superoxide dismutase on reperfusion arrhythmias and left ventricular function in patients undergoing thrombolysis for anterior wall acute myocardial infarction. Am J Cardiol 1991; **67**:765–7.

70. Flaherty JT, Pitt B, Gruber JW, Heuser RR, Rothbaum DA, Burwell LR, George BS, Kereiakes DJ, Deitchman D, Gustafson N. Recombinant human superoxide dismutase (h-SOD) fails to improve recovery of ventricular function in patients undergoing coronary angioplasty for acute myocardial infarction. Circulation 1994; **89**:1982–91.

71. Wall TC, Califf RM, Blankenship J, Talley JD, Tannenbaum M, Schwaiger M, Gacioch G, Cohen MD, Sanz M, Leimberger JD. Intravenous fluosol in the treatment of acute myocardial infarction. Results of the Thrombolysis and Angioplasty in Myocardial Infarction 9 Trial. TAMI 9 Research Group. Circulation 1994; **90**:114–20.

72. ISIS-1 investigators. Randomised trial of intravenous atenolol among 16 027 cases of suspected acute myocardial infarction: ISIS-1. First International Study of Infarct Survival Collaborative Group. Lancet 1986; **2**:57–66.

73. GISSI-3 investigators. Effects of lisinopril and transdermal glyceryl trinitrate singly and together on 6-week mortality and ventricular function after acute myocardial infarction. Gruppo Italiano per lo Studio della Sopravvivenza nell'infarto Miocardico. Lancet 1994; **343**:1115–22.

74. ISIS-4 investigators. A randomised factorial trial assessing early oral captopril, oral mononitrate, and intravenous magnesium sulphate in 58,050 patients with suspected acute myocardial infarction. ISIS-4 (Fourth International Study of Infarct Survival) Collaborative Group. Lancet 1995; **345**:669–85.

75. Secondary Prevention Reinfarction Israeli Nifedipine Trial (SPRINT). A randomized intervention trial of nifedipine in patients with acute myocardial

infarction. The Israeli Sprint Study Group. Eur Heart J 1988; **9**:354–64.

76. Multicenter Diltiazem Post Infarction Trial Research Group (MDPIT). The effect of diltiazem on mortality and reinfarction after myocardial infarction. N Engl J Med 1988; **319**:385–92.

77. Danish Study Group on Verapamil in Myocardial Infarction. Verapamil in acute myocardial infarction : the Danish Verapamil Infarction Trial I (DAVIT I). Eur Heart J 1984; **5**:516–28.

78. Danish Study Group on Verapamil in Myocardial Infarction. Effects of verapamil on mortality and major events after acute myocardial infarction: the Danish Verapamil Infarction Trial II (DAVIT II). Am J Cardiol 1990; **66**:779–85.

79. Baran KW, Nguyen M, McKendall GR, Lambrew CT, Dykstra G, Palmeri ST, Gibbons RJ, Borzak S, Sobel BE, Gourlay SG, Rundle AC, Gibson CM, Barron HV. Double-blind, randomized trial of an anti-CD18 antibody in conjunction with recombinant tissue plasminogen activator for acute myocardial infarction: limitation of myocardial infarction following thrombolysis in acute myocardial infarction (LIMIT AMI) study. Circulation 2001; **104**:2778–83.

80. Faxon DP, Gibbons RJ, Chronos NA, Gurbel PA, Sheehan F. The effect of blockade of the CD11/CD18 integrin receptor on infarct size in patients with acute myocardial infarction treated with direct angioplasty: the results of the HALT-MI study. J Am Coll Cardiol 2002; **40**:1199–204.

6

Percutaneous coronary intervention in acute ST-segment elevation of myocardial infarction

Stephen G Ellis

Angioplasty vs fibrinolytic therapy

Based upon the results of multiple randomized clinical trials in comparison with fibrinolytic therapy, primary coronary intervention, when readily available, has become the 'default mode' for management of patients seen within the first 12 hours of myocardial infarction.[1-4] This paradigm shift away from front-line use of fibrinolytic therapy is based upon individual and aggregate data summarized in meta-analysis format in Figs 6.1–6.3, as well as the results of the more recently completed DANAMI II Study.[5] In formal meta-analysis of 10 randomized trials comparing primary angioplasty with intravenous fibrinolytic therapy involving 2606 patients, Weaver and colleagues noted mortality at 30 days was 4.4% for the angioplasty treated patients compared to 6.5% for the lytic treated patients [odds ratio (OR) is 0.66; 95% confidence intervals (CI) 0.46–0.94; $p = 0.02$] (Fig. 6.1).[4] Angioplasty was also associated with a significant reduction in total stroke (0.7% vs 2.0%; $p = 0.007$), as well as the risk of recurrent myocardial infarction (MI) (Figs 6.2 and 6.3). Survival curves remained essentially parallel from 2 weeks to 6 months after treatment and the mortality benefit remained at significant at follow-up ($p = 0.04$) (Fig. 6.4).

It is perhaps disturbing that these convincing results in carefully conducted studies have not apparently been fully replicated in the community. Every and colleagues studied data from hospitals in western Washington in the United States and there appear to be minimal differences in 'risk-adjusted' mortality outcome during the first year of follow-up of over 3000 patients (Fig. 6.5).[6] Comparable results were found in the US National Registry of Myocardial Infarction (NRMI-2) (Fig. 6.6).[7] The reasons for this apparent discrepancy are probably multiple. (1) 'Risk adjustment' is never complete and there are substantial differences between the baseline characteristics of patients whom the

	Number (%)			
Study	PTCA	Lytic therapy	Odds ratio and 95% CI	p
Streptokinase				
Zijlstra et al (1993)[2]	3/152 (2.0)	11/149 (7.4)		
Ribeiro et al	3/50 (6.0)	1/50 (2.0)		
Grinfeld et al	5/54 (6.0)	6/58 (10.3)		
Zijlstra et al (1993)[2]	1/45 (2.2)	0/50		
Subtotal	**12/301 (4.0)**	**18/307 (5.9)**		0.38
t-PA				
DeWood et al	3/46 (6.5)	2/44 (4.5)		
Grines et al (1993)[1]	5/195 (2.6)	13/200 (6.5)		
Gibbons et al	2/47 (4.3)	2/56 (3.6)		
Subtotal	**10/288 (3.5)**	**17/300 (5.7)**		0.28
Accelerated t-PA				
Ribichini et al	0/41	1/42 (2.4)		
Garcia et al	3/95 (3.2)	10/94 (10.6)		
GUSTO-IIb (1997)[3]	32/565 (5.7)	40/573 (7.0)		
Subtotal	**35/701 (5.0)**	**51/709 (7.2)**		0.10
Total	**57/1290 (4.4)**	**86/1316 (6.5)**		0.02

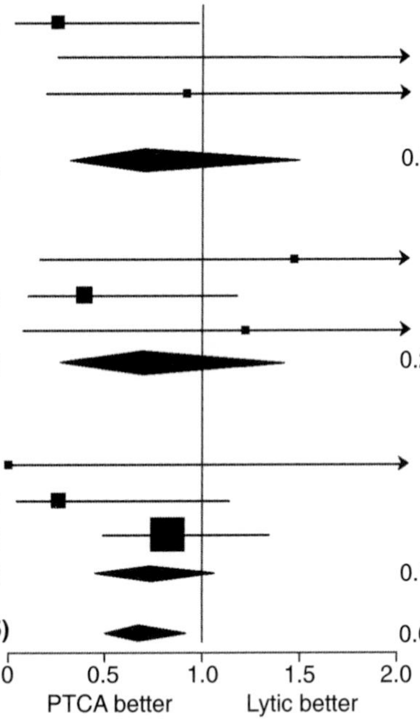

Figure 6.1

Meta-analysis of angioplasty vs fibrinolysis studies with the primary end-point of in-hospital or 30 day death. PTCA, percutaneous transluminal coronary angioplasty.

physician chooses to treat with either angioplasty or lytic therapy. (2) Operators working within the confines of clinical trials are highly selected in their experience, and technical success rates may be superior to that of the more general cardiologist. (3) Prolonged door (hospital arrival)-to-balloon times often seen in the community experience may attenuate the benefit of reperfusion with balloon angioplasty. The magnitude of this latter issue has differed in the studies in which it has been assessed. For example, Berger reporting for the results of the GUSTO-IIb study found a very considerable graded incremental risk of 30 day mortality in relation to door-to-balloon time. Patients treated within 60 min of presentation had a very low 1% mortality, whereas those treated more than 90 min after presentation had a 6.4% mortality (Fig. 6.7).[8] Conversely, the results of the NRMI-2 study show a greatly attenuated,

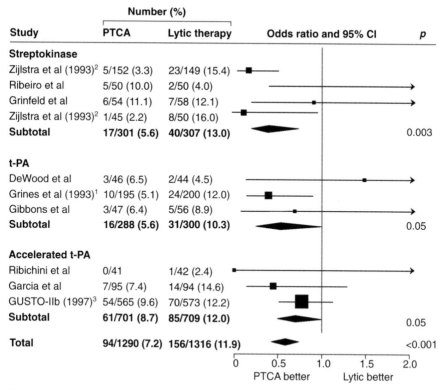

Figure 6.2

Meta-analysis of angioplasty vs fibrinolysis studies with the primary end-point of death or recurrent myocardial infarction at hospital discharge or 30 days.

but still present, relationship (Fig. 6.8).[9] These issues bear on the issue of facilitated angioplasty (see Chapter 7). On the basis of these data, the American College of Cardiology has suggested that door-to-balloon time be kept to less than 90 min.

In this context, the results of the recently presented DANAMI II study are of considerable interest, substantiating the benefit of balloon angioplasty compared to fibrinolytic therapy in patients with door-to-balloon times even as long as 3 hours.[5] In this study, in which the average patient transferred to an angioplasty site travelled 35 miles by ground transportation and not all of the angioplasty operators were highly experienced, TIMI-3 flow was established in 89% patients and the composite of death, reinfarction and stroke rates at 30 days were significantly lower with balloon angioplasty than lytics (8.0 vs 13.7%,

	Total stroke Number (%)			
Study	PTCA	Lytic therapy	Odds ratio and 95% CI	p
Streptokinase				
Zijlstra et al (1993)[2]	1/152 (0.7)	3/149 (2.0)		
Ribeiro et al	0/50	0/50		
Grinfeld et al	1/54 (1.9)	0/58		
Zijlstra et al (1993)[2]	1/45 (2.2)	2/50 (4.0)		
Subtotal	**3/301 (1.0)**	**5/307 (1.6)**		0.77
t-PA (3-4 h)				
DeWood et al	0/46	0/44		
Grines et al (1993)[1]	0/195	7/200 (3.5)		
Gibbons et al	0/47	0/56		
Subtotal	**0/288**	**7/300 (2.3)**		0.02
t-PA (accelerated)				
Ribichini et al	0/41	0/42		
Garcia et al	0/95	3/94		
GUSTO-IIb (1997)[3]	6/565 (1.1)	11/573 (1.9)		
Subtotal	**6/701 (0.86)**	**14/709 (2.0)**		0.12
Total	**9/1290 (0.7)**	**26/1316 (2.0)**		0.007

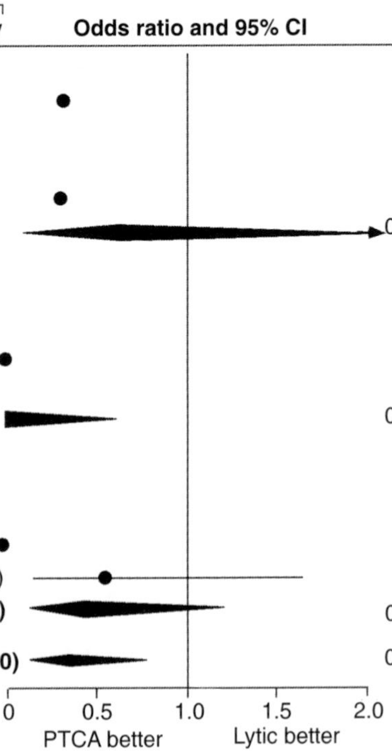

```
        0      0.5     1.0     1.5    2.0
            PTCA better      Lytic better
```

Figure 6.3
Meta-analysis of angioplasty vs fibrinolysis studies with the primary end-point of stroke at hospital discharge or 30 days.

$p = 0.0003$). While an absolute 1% reduction in 30 day mortality was seen, the principal benefits were found in a reduction in recurrent MI (6.3% vs 1.6%, $p = 0.0001$) and in a trend toward reduction of stroke (2.0% vs 1.1%).

Percutaneous transluminal coronary angioplasty (PTCA)

For patients who do receive fibrinolytic therapy and who do not do well in the early hours thereafter, acute intervention can also be contemplated. 'Rescue angioplasty', however, has not been nearly as well studied. In fact, only 505 patients have been randomized in six small studies.[10] In aggregate, PTCA performed on average of approximately 4.5 hours after initial infarct presentation for patients with demonstrated TIMI-0 or

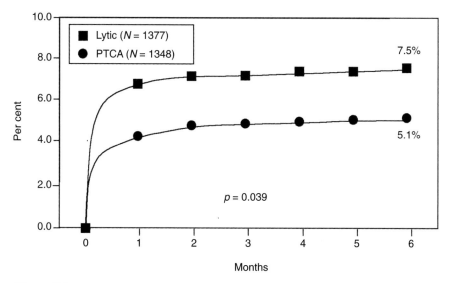

Figure 6.4
Six month survival curves in patients randomized to either PTCA or fibrinolytic therapy.

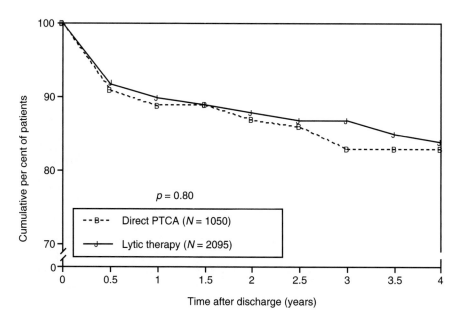

Figure 6.5
Cumulative survival among 1050 patients in the primary angioplasty group and 2095 in the fibrinolytic therapy group in the non-randomized western Washington study.

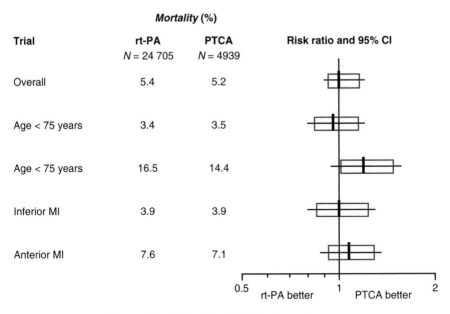

Figure 6.6

The comparison of mortality for PTCA or recombinant tissue type plasminogen activator (rt-PA) in the NRMI-2 study with subset analysis.

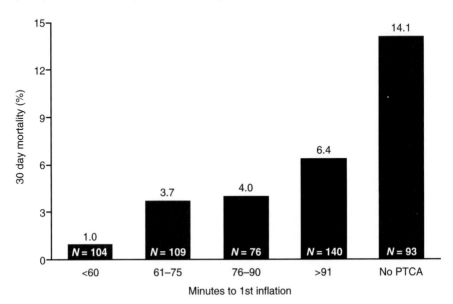

Figure 6.7

Relationship between time from study enrolment to first balloon inflation in 30 day mortality from the GUSTO-IIb study.

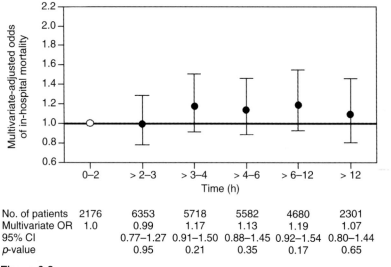

No. of patients	2176	6353	5718	5582	4680	2301
Multivariate OR	1.0	0.99	1.17	1.13	1.19	1.07
95% CI		0.77–1.27	0.91–1.50	0.88–1.45	0.92–1.54	0.80–1.44
p-value		0.95	0.21	0.35	0.17	0.65

Figure 6.8

Relationship between time intervals of door-to-balloon time and mortality in the NRMI-2 study.

TIMI-1 flow appeared to reduce early severe heart failure (3.8% vs 11.7%; $p = 0.04$), improve survival over 1 year in patients with moderate to large MI (92% vs 87%; $p = 0.001$) and possibly reduce early repeat MI (4.3% vs 11.3%; $p = 0.08$) (Fig. 6.9). Given that the largest study assessing this issue required patients to have anterior wall infarction that could be treated within 8 hours of infarct onset, it is difficult to extrapolate these data to patients with smaller infarcts or those who might be treated later.[11] Assessment of a possible benefit of PTCA for patients with TIMI-2 flow after fibrinolysis is even further hampered by the small number of patients randomly assigned. Of the 137 patients in total randomized in two studies, there was no apparent benefit of angioplasty with regard to death or recurrent infarction, but both studies suggested an improvement in left ventricular function at follow-up.[10] The question as to whether coronary intervention has any utility for patients with patent coronary arteries after fibrinolytic therapy (TIMI-2 or TIMI-3 flow) has not been formally addressed since the mid 1980s when three small studies demonstrated conclusively that balloon angioplasty as it was performed at that time period had no clinical benefit and in fact was associated with a marginally statistically significant adverse effect on mortality (3.6% vs 6.3%; $p = 0.05$).[12–14] These studies, with the exception of the TAMI-1 study did not appreciate the clinical significance between TIMI-2 and TIMI-3 flow; hence one cannot be certain of what proportion of patients in these studies actually had TIMI-3 flow before angioplasty.[12,15] Notably, however, with advances in both mechanical and adjunctive pharmacological

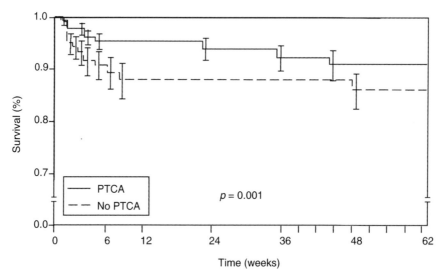

Figure 6.9

Long-term follow-up from the only two studies of rescue angioplasty providing such follow-up.

therapy applied now in the setting of rescue angioplasty, results appear to be considerably better; hence the merit of intervention in this setting must be considered conjectural.[10,16]

Cardiogenic shock

The special situation of patients presenting in cardiogenic shock from acute myocardial infarction (AMI) should be considered separately as these patients were excluded from the aforementioned randomized trials. Non-randomized studies have clearly demonstrated that percutaneous intervention for patients with cardiogenic shock results in TIMI-3 flow rates only slightly less than that achieved in more stable patients. The results of the SHOCK study, the only large randomized trial of revascularization in shock, strongly suggest that early emergency revascularization in patients presenting with shock complicating AMI achieve a survival advantage when compared to more conservative therapy, at least for patients under the age of 75.[17] Of patients randomized to revascularization, approximately two-thirds had angioplasty and one-third had bypass surgery. Coronary disease was more extensive in the later group but the 30 day mortalities did not differ (45.3% and 42.1%, respectively). Non-randomized data from the Cleveland Clinic suggests that the benefit of percutaneous revascularization in this trial may be underestimated relative to what might be achieved with more contemporary therapy. In that study, after an average of 2 years follow-up the mortality rates for patients in cardiogenic shock treated with stent plus abciximab, stent only, PTCA plus abciximab, and PTCA alone were 33%, 43%, 61% and 68%, respectively (p = 0.028).[18]

The optimal technical approach to intervention in the setting of AMI continues to be debated. Clearly, one should proceed expeditiously to the catheterization laboratory with an experienced team, stabilize the patient rapidly, utilizing a balloon pump if necessary, and open the culprit vessel promptly. Patients with left main occlusion need not be avoided, although their in-hospital mortality remains high (although if they survived a hospital discharge, intermediate term survival is actually quite good).[19] Only in the setting of cardiogenic shock should more than the culprit lesion be treated, although with stents and intravenous glycoprotein (GP) IIb/IIIa inhibitors improving the safety of the overall approach, the safety and efficacy of treating multiple lesions has begun to be re-examined.[20]

Stenting vs balloon angioplasty

The merits of stenting as opposed to only balloon angioplasty only in suitable vessels has been examined in a number of trials, with generally concordant results typified by the largest and most recently published CADILLAC trial: no improvement in survival, a modest benefit in reduction of reinfarction or early urgent revascularization and a highly significant reduction in late target vessel revascularization (Fig. 6.10).[21] Some have argued that many of these studies, in particular CADILLAC, enrolled only low-risk patients; hence the results are not entirely representative. Non-randomized data do suggest a potential benefit of stenting in higher-risk patients,[18] but it is on the basis of cumulative results to 6 months that most agree that stents should be placed when possible. The further potential benefits of heparin-coated or antirestenotic-coated stents remain to be fully evaluated but are likely to further improve the long-term results.[22] Aspirin, unfractionated heparin, and now the thienopyridine adenosine 5′-diphosphate (ADP) inhibitor clopidogrel form the current backbone of adjunctive pharmacological therapy utilized to optimize vessel patency in this setting. Beta blockers, angiotensin-converting enzyme (ACE) inhibitors and statins should be added as early as possible. The potential merit of GP IIb/IIIa antagonists remains debated. In the largest evaluation, the CADILLAC trial found a 1.3% absolute improvement in composite 30 day study outcome with abciximab and stenting compared to stenting alone, but this was driven entirely by ischaemic target vessel revascularization and there was absolutely no difference in death or reinfarction (Fig. 6.10). Two smaller randomized trials have found a larger clinical benefit with abciximab (Fig. 6.11), as well as an improvement in follow-up ejection fraction (Fig. 6.12), presumably due

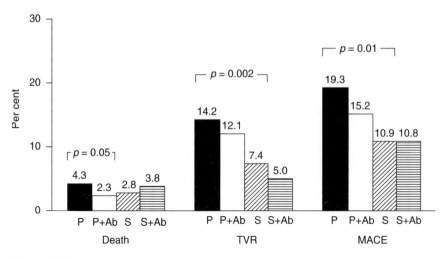

Figure 6.10
Principal 30 day outcomes from the CADILLAC study randomizing patients with AMI to angioplasty (P) or stenting (S), and abciximab (Ab) or no abciximab. MACE, major adverse cardiovascular event; TVR, target vessel revascularization.

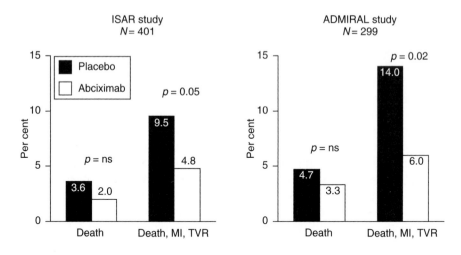

Figure 6.11
Early clinical outcomes in the ADMIRAL and ISAR studies of primary stenting with or without adjunctive abciximab. ns, not significant; MI, myocardial infarction; TVR, target vessel revascularization.

to an improvement in microvascular flow.[23,24] In aggregate, then, it is probably prudent to utilize these agents in all but patients at highest risk of bleeding. The potential merit of using emboli protection devices in this setting is just beginning to be investigated.

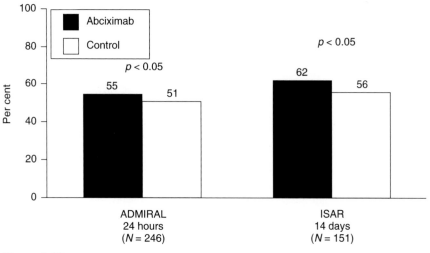

Figure 6.12

Early left ventricular (LV) ejection fraction in patients from the ISAR and ADMIRAL studies randomizing patients with AMI undergoing coronary stenting to abciximab or no abciximab.

Exactly how long to wait for non-invasive evidence of reperfusion, and how to assess that parameter are questions that complicate the use of rescue angioplasty. Clearly, ST-segment resolution at 60 and 90 min does correlate with the approved 30 day survival, probably reflecting both the area of insult and vessel patency.[25] Optimal outcomes are seen with > 70% resolution of summed ST-segment elevation compared to baseline.[25] Clinical judgement is required to integrate this information with the patient's presentation and degree of haemodynamic stability, but generally, if one is to actively pursue a strategy of rescue angioplasty, arrangements for urgent transfer for cardiac catheterization should be made in the patient with an apparent large infarct who does not have at least 50% ST-segment resolution and some degree of haemodynamic stabilization by approximately 60 min after the institution of fibrinolytic therapy.

Conclusion

Despite advances in the pharmacological approach to coronary reperfusion in this setting, including the combined use of fibrinolytic agents and glycoprotein IIb/IIIa inhibitors, restoration of TIMI-3 flow remains superior with mechanical intervention and hence it is the preferred therapy for virtually all patients with acute ST-segment elevation myocardial infarction. If fibrinolytic therapy needs to be utilized because of lack of access to mechanical reperfusion, it is of course preferable in most patients to more conservative management, but probably should be supplemented with the concept of rescue angioplasty for patients with large infarcts who appear not be achieving the early benefits of reperfusion therapy.

References

1. Grines CL, Browne KF, Marco J, Rothbaum D, Stone GW, O'Keefe J, Overlie P, Donohue B, Chelliah N, Timmis GC. A comparison of immediate angioplasty with thrombolytic therapy for acute myocardial infarction. The Primary Angioplasty in Myocardial Infarction Study Group. N Engl J Med 1993; **328**:673–9.

2. Zijlstra F, de Boer JM, Hoorntje JC, Reiffers S, Reiber JH, Suryapranata H. A comparison of immediate coronary angioplasty with intravenous streptokinase in acute myocardial infarction. N Engl J Med 1993; **328**:680–4.

3. GUSTO IIb Angioplasty Substudy investigators. A clinical trial comparing primary coronary angioplasty with tissue plasminogen activator for acute myocardial infarction. N Engl J Med 1997; **336**:1621–8.

4. Weaver DW, Simes RJ, Betriu A, Grines C, Zijlstra F, Eulogio G, Grinfeld L, Gibbons RJ, Ribeiro EE, DeWood MA, Ribichini F. Comparison of primary coronary angioplasty and intravenous thrombolytic therapy for acute myocardial infarction: A quantitative review. JAMA 1997; **278**:2093–8.

5. Anderson HR. The results of the DANAMI II Study as presented at the American College of Cardiology meeting, Atlanta, GA, USA, 20 March, 2002.

6. Every NR, Parsons LS, Hlatky M, Nartin JS, Weaver WD for the Myocardial Infarction Triage and Intervention Investigators: A comparison of thrombolytic therapy with primary coronary angioplasty for acute myocardial infarction. N Engl J Med 1996; **335**:1253–60.

7. Tiefenbrunn AJ, Chandra NC, French WJ, Gore JM, Rogers WJ. Clinical experience with primary percutaneous transluminal coronary angioplasty compared with alteplase (recombinant tissue-type plasminogen activator) in patients with acute myocardial infarction. A report from the Second National Registry of Myocardial Infarction (NRMI-2). Circulation 1998; **31**:1240–5.

8. Berger PB, Ellis SG, Holmes DR Jr, Granger CB, Criger DA, Betriu A, Topol EJ, Califf RM for the GUSTO-II Investigators. Relationship between delay in performing direct coronary angioplasty and early clinical outcome in patients with acute myocardial infarction: Results from the Global Use of Strategies to Open Occluded Arteries in Acute Coronary Syndromes (GUSTO-IIb) Trial. Circulation 1999; **100**:14–20.

9. Cannon CP, Gibson CM, Lambrew CT, Shoultz DA, Levy D, French WJ, Gore JM, Weaver WD, Rogers WJ, Tiefenbrunn AJ. Relationship of symptom-onset-to-balloon time and door-to-balloon time with mortality in patients undergoing angioplasty for acute myocardial infarction. JAMA 2000; **2083**:2941–7.

10. Ellis SG, Ribeiro da Silva E, Spaulding CM, Nobuyoshi M, Weiner B, Talley JD. Review of immediate angioplasty after fibrinolytic therapy for acute myocardial infarction: Insights from the RESCUE I, RESCUE II, and other contemporary clinical experiences. Am Heart J 2000; **139**:1046–53.

11. Ellis SG, Ribeiro da Silva E, Heyndrickx G, Talley JD, Cernigliaro C, Steg G, Spaulding C, Nobuyoshi M, Erbel R, Vassanelli C, Topol EJ for the RESCUE Investigators. Randomized comparison of rescue angioplasty with conservative management of patients with early failure of thrombolysis for acute anterior myocardial infarction. Circulation 1994; **90**:2280–4.

12. Topol EJ, Califf RM, George BS, Kereiakes DJ, Abbottsmith CV, Candela RJ, Lee KL, Pitt B, Stack RS, O'Neil WW. Thrombolysis and Angioplasty in Myocardial Infarction Study Group. A randomized trial of immediate versus delayed elective angioplasty after intravenous tissue plasminogen activator in acute myocardial infarction. N Engl J Med 1987; **317**:581–8.

13. TIMI Study Group. Immediate vs. delayed catheterization and angioplasty following thrombolytic therapy for acute myocardial infarction: TIMI IIA results. JAMA 1998; **260**:2849–58.

14. Simoons ML, Arnold AE, Betriu A, de Bono DP, Col J, Dougherty FC, Von Essen R, Lambertz H, Lubsen J, Meier B. Thrombolysis with tissue plasminogen activator in acute myocardial infarction: no additional benefit from immediate percutaneous coronary angioplasty. Lancet 1988; **1**: 197–202.

15. Ellis SG, Lincoff AM, George BS, Kereiakes DJ, Ohman EM, Krucoff MW, Califf RM, Topol EJ, the Thrombolysis and Angioplasty In Myocardial Infarction (TAMI) Study Group. Randomized evaluation of coronary angioplasty for early TIMI 2 flow after thrombolytic therapy for the treatment of acute myocardial infarction—a new look at an old study. Coron Arter Dis 1994; **5**:611–15.

16. Ohman EM, Kleiman NS, Gacioch G et al. Combined accelerated tissue-plasminogen activator and platelet glycoprotein IIb/IIIa integrin receptor blockade with Integrilin in acute myocardial infarction. Results of a randomized, placebo-controlled, dose-ranging trial. IMPACT-AMI Investigators. Circulation 1997; **95**:846–54.

17. Hochman JS, Sleeper LA, Webb JG, Sanborn TA, White HD, Talley JD, Buller CE, Jacobs AK, Slater JN, Col J, McKinlay SM, LeJemtel TH for the SHOCK Investigators. Early revascularization in acute myocardial infarction complicated by cardiogenic shock. N Engl J Med 1999; **341**:625–34.

18. Chan AW, Chew DP, Bhatt DL, Moliterno DJ, Topol EJ, Ellis SG. Long-term mortality benefit with the combination of stents and abciximab for cardiogenic shock complicating acute myocardial infarction. Am J Cardiol 2002; **89**:132–6.

19. Marso SP, Steg G, Plokker T, Holmes D, Park S-J, Kosuga K, Tamai H, Macaya C, Moses J, White H, Verstraete SFC, Ellis SG. Catheter-based reperfusion of unprotected left main stenosis during an acute myocardial infarction (the ULTIMA experience). Am J Cardiol 1999; **83**:1513–17.

20. Roe MT, Cura FA, Joski PS, Garcia E, Guetta V, Kereiakes DJ, Zijlstra F, Brodie BR, Grines CL, Ellis SG. Initial experience with multivessel percutaneous coronary intervention during mechanical reperfusion for acute myocardial infarction. Am J Cardiol 2001; **88**:170–3.

21. Stone GW, Grines CL, Cox DA, Garcia E, Tcheng JE, Griffin JJ, Guagliumi G, Stuckey T, Turco M, Carroll JD, Rutherford BD, Lansky AJ for the Controlled Abciximab and Device Investigation to Lower Late Angioplasty Complications (CADILLAC) Investigators. Comparison of angioplasty with stenting, with or without abciximab, in acute myocardial infarction. N Engl J Med 2002; **346**:957–66.

22. Fajadet J, Perin M, Ban Hayashi E, Colombo A, Schuler G, Barragan P, Bode C, Sousa JE, Morice MC, Serruys PW. 210-Day follow-up of the RAVEL study: A randomized study with the sirolimus-eluting Bx VELOCITY™ balloon-expandable stent in the treatment of patients with de novo native coronary artery lesions. J Am Coll Cardiol 2002; **39**:20A.

23. Montalescot G, Barragan P, Wittenberg O, Ecollan P, Elhadad S, Villain P, Boulenc JM, Morice MC, Millard L, Pansieri M, Choussat R, Pinton P, ADMIRAL Investigators. Abciximab before direct angioplasty and stenting in myocardial infarction regarding acute and long-term follow-up. Platelet glycoprotein, IIb/IIIa inhibition with coronary stenting for acute myocardial infarction. N Engl J Med 2001; **344**: 1895–903.

24. Neumann FJ, Kastrati A, Miethke T, Pogatsa-Murray G, Mehilli J, Valina C, Jogethaei N, da Costa CP, Wagner H, Schömig A. Treatment of *Chlamydia pneumoNiae* infection with roxithromycin and effect on neointima proliferation after coronary stent placement (ISAR-3): a randomized, double-blind, placebo-controlled trial. Lancet 2001; **357**:2085–9.

25. Schröder R, Wegscheider K, Schröder K, Dissmann R, Meyer-Sabellek W. Extent of early ST segment elevation resolution: a strong predictor of outcome in patients with acute myocardial infarction and a sensitive measure to compare thrombolytic regiments. A substudy of the International Joint Efficacy Comparison of Thrombolytics. J Am Coll Cardiol 1995; **26**:1657–64.

7
Pre-hospital fibrinolytic therapy

Eric Boersma

Time is muscle—and muscle is life

Experimental and clinical data support the concept that an acute myocardial infarction (AMI) usually occurs as a result of a sudden thrombotic obstruction of the infarct-related coronary artery, superimposed on a ruptured atherosclerotic plaque.[1] The duration of the coronary occlusion, and the extent of collateral circulation are the main determinants of infarct size in pigs, dogs, cats and other animals.[2-7] In animals with a coronary collateral circulation similar to that of humans an occlusion persisting for 15–30 minutes generally does not lead to significant myocardial damage. Thus, necrosis can be prevented provided reperfusion is achieved within this period. A small area of necrosis usually occurs with reperfusion after 45 min of occlusion, while the mid-endocardial and sub-endocardial zones are still viable. Longer durations of coronary occlusion result in progressive growth of the infarction and reduction of the amount of salvageable myocardium (Fig. 7.1). At 90 min the extent of cell death involves 40–50% of the area at risk; less than half of the jeopardized myocardium remains viable at that time point. Six hours after the onset of continuous ischaemia the area at risk is fully infarcted such that myocardial salvage will be minimal.

In humans, the thrombotic event frequently consists of multiple cycles of temporary occlusion and reperfusion. The degree of chest pain varies among patients, so that it is often difficult to determine the exact duration of the coronary occlusion. Nevertheless, data indicate that evolution of (enzymatically detectable) infarct size over time in humans shows a pattern similar to that in animals. In a study involving 1334 myocardial infarction (MI) patients, the cumulative release of myocardial α-hydroxybutyrate dehydrogenase during the first 72 hours after infarction was comparatively small in those treated within 1 hour from onset of symptoms (Fig. 7.2).[8] A very steep increase in the rate of enzyme release was noted between 1 and 2 hours of treatment delay, whereas the increase was relatively small thereafter.

The value of fibrinolytic therapy in patients with evolving MI is well documented. Timely fibrinolytic therapy interrupts the process of evolving myocardial necrosis, which results in salvage of viable myocardium,

111

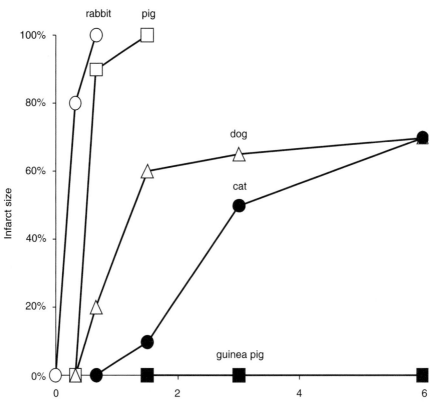

Figure 7.1

Development of infarct size as percentage of the infarct size that would occur when the coronary artery is permanently occluded in various animal species. Adapted from DeWood et al (1980).[2]

preservation of left ventricular (LV) function, and consequently, improved survival. A meta-analysis of large randomized trials that compared fibrinolytic therapy with control (including almost 60 000 patients) showed an absolute mortality reduction of about 30/1000 patients presenting within 6 hours, and of about 20/1000 patients presenting between 6 and 12 hours from onset of symptoms.[9] A more detailed analysis of the relation between treatment delay and treatment effect, which also included data from smaller trials, indicated that the mortality reduction by fibrinolytic therapy was greatest among patients presenting within 1 hour from symptom onset.[10] The proportional mortality reduction in this group was as high as 50% (Fig. 7.3), whereas the absolute mortality reduction was estimated at 65/1000 patients treated (Fig. 7.4). Fibrinolytic treatment that is initiated within 2 hours results in a significantly higher proportional

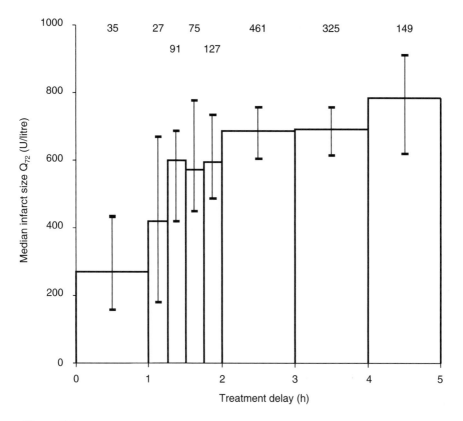

Figure 7.2

Effect of delay of fibrinolytic treatment on infarct size. Numbers above columns are number
of patients. Columns represent mean values; vertical bars represent 95% confidence
intervals. Q_{72}, cumulative activity of myocardial α-hydroxybutyrate dehydrogenase
released per litre of plasma during the first 24 h after acute myocardial infarction.
Adapted from Hermens et al (1992).[8]

mortality reduction than later treatment (45% vs 20%), indicating that most
benefit of fibrinolysis can be obtained during the ongoing process of
myocardial cell death. Therefore, to realize the full potential of the life-
saving effects of fibrinolytic therapy, treatment should be initiated as soon
as possible after symptom onset, preferably within the first 1 to 2 hours.
Unfortunately, to date, only a minority of MI patients (5–10%) receive such
early fibrinolysis.

Treatment delay in clinical practice, and the need for pre-hospital triage and therapy

The time that expires between the onset of chest pain, which is supposed
to coincide with the coronary obstruction, and the initiation of fibrinolytic

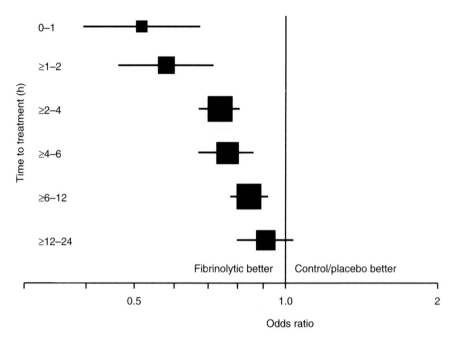

Figure 7.3

Proportional effect of fibrinolytic therapy on 35 day mortality according to treatment delay. Data are derived from all 22 trials conducted between 1983 and 1993 that included at least 100 patients who were randomized between fibrinolytic therapy or control.[10] Odds ratios, plotted with their 95% CI on a log scale, are significantly different over the six groups (Breslow-Day test, p = 0.001). The areas of the black squares are proportional to the amount of statistical information. Adapted from Boersma et al (1996).[10]

therapy consists of three main components. First, the patient needs time to recognize the cardiac nature and severity of the problems, and to seek medical help. Unfortunately, most patients fail to react rapidly to symptoms. Data from (inter)national registries of myocardial infarctions (MIs) in the United States and in Europe indicate that about 50% of patients who are eligible for fibrinolytic therapy do not report their symptoms within 3 hours.[11,12] Another 25% do not arrive at the hospital emergency department until 6 hours or later, including 10% who arrive 12 hours or later, a period in which fibrinolytic therapy has lost its life-saving capacity.

The second component of total treatment delay is the time needed for transportation to the hospital. Depending on the local infrastructure, the distance to the nearest hospital, and the time of day (traffic jams), the transport delay may vary considerably.[13–15] It usually takes 10–15 min before arrival of the ambulance at the patient's home. Another 10–15 min is needed for preparation, and again another 10–15 min for the actual transport.

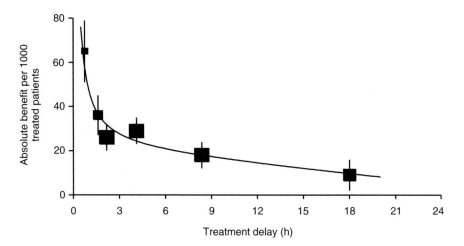

Figure 7.4

Absolute 35 day mortality reduction vs treatment delay. The regression line is fitted within data that are derived from all 22 trials conducted between 1983 and 1993 that included at least 100 patients who were randomized between fibrinolytic therapy or control.[10] Black squares: average effects in six time-to-treatment groups (the areas of these squares are inversely proportional to the variance of absolute benefit described). Adapted from Boersma et al (1996).[10]

The third component of treatment delay is the time needed in-hospital for nursing, initial evaluation by an emergency room physician, ECG recording and interpretation, laboratory testing, further evaluation by an experienced staff cardiologist, and transport from the emergency room to the coronary care unit where therapy is subsequently administered. Data from a broad spectrum of European clinical practices demonstrate that the time needed for in-hospital decision making is considerable: the median time from arrival at the emergency room to fibrinolytic therapy is as long as 60 min.[12] Guidelines recommend that in-hospital treatment delay (door-to-needle time) should be less than 20 min.[16] In clinical practice, however, only about 25% of patients who are treated with a fibrinolytic agent receive that agent within this time period. Available data from other parts of the world show similar worrisome results.

One might expect that the increasing literature on the importance of early fibrinolytic therapy in acute myocardial infarction (AMI) would have resulted in decreasing treatment delays over the past few years. This, however, seems not to be the case. The mean delay from onset of symptoms to the initiation of fibrinolytic therapy in mega-trials of MI patients (with similar inclusion criteria) has hardly changed since the beginning of the 1990s (Fig. 7.5). In fact, treatment delays have slightly increased since that time, with a mean value of 165 min in GUSTO-I (1993) and 198 min in HERO-2 (2001).[17,18]

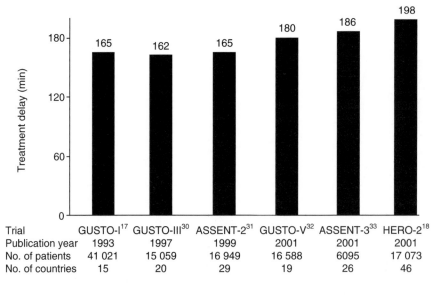

Trial	GUSTO-I[17]	GUSTO-III[30]	ASSENT-2[31]	GUSTO-V[32]	ASSENT-3[33]	HERO-2[18]
Publication year	1993	1997	1999	2001	2001	2001
No. of patients	41 021	15 059	16 949	16 588	6095	17 073
No. of countries	15	20	29	19	26	46

Figure 7.5

Mean time from symptom onset to fibrinolytic treatment in mega-trials (1993–2001) of myocardial infarction patients. All trials randomized patients within 6 hours from onset of symptoms.

How can these results be improved? First, the public, and in particular patients with known coronary disease, should be made aware of the symptoms of a 'heart attack' and the value of immediate therapy. In all communities, early warning systems should be encouraged. Patients should be offered an easy and rapid access to medical therapy. Studies in different communities have shown that greater awareness does indeed reduce the patient delay. Second, a treatment strategy should be implemented that aims at a rapid and accurate triage at the patient's home, and that allows for—after myocardial infarction is confirmed—immediate fibrinolytic therapy by a general practitioner or paramedic. Such pre-hospital diagnosis and treatment strategies have been evaluated in a number of randomized clinical trials. Third, in each hospital a registry should be kept of treatment delays, and specific measures taken whenever these delays get out of the hand. In the presence of extensive ST-segment elevation on the ECG no time should be lost with consultation. The emergency physician, and even nurses (if no physician is immediately available) should have a mandate to initiate therapy immediately.

Randomized trials of pre-hospital vs in-hospital fibrinolysis

There are eight randomized trials that compared pre-hospital with in-hospital fibrinolytic therapy.[13–15,19–23] Although most of these studies were too small to show statistical significance, together they provide compelling evidence that pre-hospital fibrinolysis is feasible, safe and effective, on the understanding that conditions are fulfilled with regard to a proper diagnosis and (relative) contraindications.

The European Myocardial Infarction Project (EMIP) is the largest such trial. EMIP was undertaken during 1988–1992 in 163 cardiological practices in 15 European countries and Canada.[13] Patients with chest pain suggestive of MI and lasting for at least 30 min, or pain lasting for less than 30 min but still present and not responsive to nitrates, who were seen within 6 hours from the onset of symptoms were eligible if the ECG confirmed the diagnosis of MI. Classical electrocardiographic requirements were applied: ST-segment elevation ≥1 mm in ≥2 limb leads and/or elevation ≥2 mm in ≥2 precordial leads. Excluded were patients who were at increased risk of bleeding complications (Table 7.1), and patients who were known or suspected to be pregnant. There was no upper age limit. Eligible patients who gave their consent to participate were randomly (and double-blind) assigned to immediate fibrinolytic therapy (anistreplase) followed by placebo in the hospital, or placebo before admission followed by anistreplase in the hospital. Pre-hospital screening, diagnosis (including ECG interpretation) and initiation of study medication was performed by ambulance attendants, nurses and accompanying physicians.

Table 7.1 Inclusion criteria and exclusion criteria that are applied in three major randomized clinical trials of pre-hospital vs in-hospital fibrinolysis.

	EMIP[13]	MITI[14]	GREAT[15]
Inclusion criteria			
Minimal duration of symptoms	30 min	–	20 min
Maximal duration of symptoms	6 h	6 h	4 h
No relief by nitroglycerin	×	–	–
ECG findings	×	×	–
Exclusion criteria			
Cardiac massage	×	–	×
Blood pressure	>200/120	>180/120	>200/–
Known bleeding disorder	×	–	×
Pregnancy / menstruation	×	–	×
Use of oral anticoagulants	×	–	×
Previous thrombolysis	–	–	×
History of stroke	×	×	×
Recent history of:			
– Major trauma	×	×	×
– Surgery	×	×	×
– Percutaneous coronary intervention	×	–	–
– Gastroduodenal ulcer or blood loss	×	–	×

EMIP, European Myocardial Infarction Project; MITI, Myocardial Infarction Triage and Intervention trial; GREAT, Grampian Region Early Anistreplase Trial.

The primary study end-point was death from all causes by 30 days. According to the design, 10 000 patients should have been randomized to detect a 15% reduction in the primary end-point in favour of pre-hospital fibrinolysis, but the trial was terminated prematurely because of lack of funding. Finally, 5469 patients were enrolled. The median time from symptom onset to treatment in patients randomized to pre-hospital fibrinolysis was 130 min, compared to 190 min in the in-hospital treated group. The median time gained with pre-hospital treatment was 55 min. The diagnosis of MI was confirmed in hospital in 90% of patients. Another 7% of patients had an acute coronary syndrome, but MI could not be confirmed. Two percent of patients were diagnosed as non-cardiac disease; 21 patients (0.4%) had pericarditis. The incidence of ventricular fibrillation, shock and symptomatic hypotension during transportation was higher in patients randomized to pre-hospital fibrinolysis, but patients randomized to in-hospital treatment had a higher incidence of these complications during hospital stay (Table 7.2). As a result, there was no difference in the overall incidence between the two groups. Thirty day mortality was 9.6% in patients randomized to pre-hospital fibrinolysis and 11.1% in in-hospital fibrinolysis, implying a 13% relative mortality reduction, and a 1.5% absolute mortality reduction.

The Myocardial Infarction Triage and Intervention (MITI) trial was performed during 1989–1991, and involved 19 hospitals in the area of Seattle, Washington, United States.[14] Patients aged 75 years or younger who had symptoms suggestive of AMI, chest pain for less than 6 hours, and no risk factors for serious bleeding (Table 7.1), were further evaluated for inclusion in the trial. A 12-lead ECG was derived by a paramedic, using a portable, computer-interpreted ECG system (Marquette Electronics), and subsequently transmitted to the emergency department of the paramedic base hospital. A physician in the emergency department reviewed the clinical and ECG findings, and made the final treatment decision. Patients who consented were randomly allocated to receive either pre- or in-hospital fibrinolytic (alteplase, rt-PA) treatment. No placebo was given to patients randomized to in-hospital treatment. The primary end-point of the trial was a ranked composite score that combined death, stroke, major bleeding, and infarct size.

MITI enrolled 360 patients. The median time from symptom onset to treatment was 77 min for the patients allocated to pre-hospital treatment and 110 min for those allocated to in-hospital treatment. The median time gained with pre-hospital treatment was 33 min. MI was confirmed in 98% of patients; 1% of patients had no enzyme elevation, and were diagnosed as unstable angina; 1 patient (0.3%) had pericarditis. The composite outcome score was similar for both arms of the trial. Mortality rates were 5.7% and 8.1% in patients randomized to pre- and in-hospital treatment, respectively.

Table 7.2 Major complications according allocated treatment arm in three randomized clinical trials of pre-hospital vs in-hospital fibrinolysis.

	EMIP[13]		MITI[14]		GREAT[15]	
	Pre	In	Pre	In	Pre	In
N	2750	2719	163	148	175	185
Pre-hospital						
Death	1.3	0.9	1.8	3.4	–	–
Ventricular fibrillation	2.5	1.6	–	–	–	–
Cardiac arrest	1.6	1.2	0	2.7	<1	<1
Pulmonary oedema	2.3	2.3	–	–	12	
Shock	6.3	3.9	1.2	1.4	3	
Stroke	0.1	0	0	0	–	–
In-hospital						
Death	8.4	10.2	4.9	8.1	–	–
Ventricular fibrillation	11.1	13.9	–	–	–	–
Cardiac arrest	12.0	15.0	1.2	2.0	–	–
Pulmonary oedema	23.0	24.9			–	–
Shock	24.6	26.5	–	–	–	–
Stroke	3.0	3.0	0.6	0.6	–	–
Total						
Death	9.7	11.1	6.7	11.5	5.3	11.9
Ventricular fibrillation	13.6	15.5	–	–	–	–
Cardiac arrest	13.6	16.2	1.2	4.7	–	–
Pulmonary oedema	25.3	27.2			–	–
Shock	30.9	30.4	–	–	–	–
Stroke	3.1	3.0	0.6	0.6	2.3	1.1

EMIP, European Myocardial Infarction Project; MITI, Myocardial Infarction Triage and Intervention trial; GREAT, Grampian Region Early Anistreplase Trial. Pre, randomized to pre-hospital fibrinolytic treatment; In, randomized to in-hospital fibrinolytic treatment.

The Grampian Region Early Anistreplase Trial (GREAT), which was undertaken during 1988–1991, involved 29 rural general practices in the region of Grampian, Scotland.[15] These practices are located in small villages at a distance of 26–100 km (16–62 miles) from Aberdeen, the closest city with adequate hospital facilities. Entry to the trial was a strong clinical suspicion of AMI by the general practitioner (GP). Symptoms suggestive of MI had to have been present for at least 20 min, but no longer than 4 hours (because for ethical reasons it had to be possible for the patients to get to Aberdeen within 6 hours after symptom onset). The GP was equipped with an electrocardiograph and he/she was required to record an ECG. However, no formal ECG criteria were applied for study entry. Excluded were patients with a suspected high risk of major bleeding complications (Table 7.1). Patients who agreed to participate were randomly assigned to immediate fibrinolytic therapy (anistreplase) followed by placebo in the hospital, or placebo before admission followed by anistreplase in the hospital. Randomization was double-blind. The primary end-point of the trial was in accordance with the main purpose: to study the feasibility and safety of pre-hospital fibrinolytic therapy. Efficacy (i.e. mortality reduction) was a secondary end-point.

Altogether, 311 patients participated in GREAT. The median times from symptom onset to home and hospital treatment were 105 min and 240 min, respectively. This difference was apparently larger than in EMIP and MITI, and can partly be explained by the large distance from the Grampian region to Aberdeen: the journey time was estimated at approximately 45 min. However, also the in-hospital delays (door-to-needle time) were considerable: about 90 min. The proportion of trial patients with a final, hospital discharge diagnosis of MI was 78%, importantly lower than in EMIP and MITI; 11% of patients were classified as having ischaemic heart disease (but no infarction), whereas another 9% had aspecific chest pain. It should be realized, in this respect, that in GREAT no expert support was given to GPs for the interpretation of the qualifying ECG. Inadequate interpretation of ECGs result in a relatively low specificity of the diagnostic 'system'. Hospital discharge mortality rates were 6.7% and 11.5% in patients allocated to pre- and in-hospital fibrinolytic treatment, respectively.

In summary, an apparent reduction in treatment delay can be reached if the diagnosis of MI and subsequent initiation of fibrinolytic therapy can be displaced from the hospital to the patient's home. More importantly, the strategy of pre-hospital triage and treatment enables fibrinolytic treatment within the first golden hour in a considerable proportion of patients. In the combined data of all randomized trials of pre- versus in-hospital fibrinolysis a 1 hour time gain was noted: the median delays were 125 min and 186 min, respectively. This 1 hour earlier treatment was associated with a benefit of approximately 20 lives per 1000 patients treated (Fig. 7.6). Indeed, it is a paying option to bring the treatment to the patient.

Benefits and risks in pre-hospital fibrinolysis

The safety of pre-hospital fibrinolysis strongly depends on the possibilities of correct diagnosis in the pre-hospital setting. Because of the—be it moderate—risk of severe, life-threatening bleeding complications associated with fibrinolytic agents, inappropriate treatment should be avoided in patients with indicative symptoms, but without developing an infarction. A correctly interpreted ECG is essential in this respect (remember the GREAT results). The occurrence of ST-segment deviation (ST-segment elevation and concomitant depression) on the ECG is the most specific electrocardiographic measure for confirmation of evolving myocardial

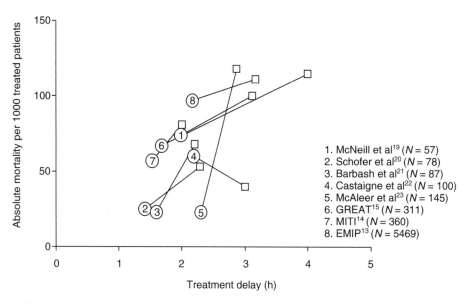

Figure 7.6

Mortality at 35 days in randomized studies comparing pre-hospital (circles) with in-hospital (squares) fibrinolytic therapy. All trials (except Castaigne et al) showed a trend favouring pre-hospital fibrinolysis. The regression line (bold, weighted by the number of patients included in the mortality result) was mainly determined by the EMIP study. Adapted from Boersma et al (1996).[10]

infarction.[24] The percentage of MIs to be confirmed (sensitivity) and of non-infarctions to be excluded (specificity) is related to the selected thresholds for ST deviation. The choice of these thresholds for pre-hospital fibrinolysis is arbitrary and depends on the perceived benefits of appropriate and risks of inappropriate treatment. Figure 7.7 demonstrates the sensitivity and specificity for MI in relation to thresholds of ST deviation as observed in a study of 1072 consecutive patients presenting within 6 hours from the onset of chest pain suggestive of acute cardiac pathology.[25] These patients were transported by the ambulance service in the region of Rotterdam, The Netherlands. Ambulance nurses derived an ECG prior to hospital admission. Note that the classical criteria for in-hospital electrocardiographic confirmation of evolving myocardial infarction (ST-segment elevation ≥1 mm in ≥2 limb leads and/or elevation ≥2 mm in ≥2 precordial leads) were satisfied in 49 out of 701 patients without a final diagnosis of MI, implying a specificity of 93% of the ECG in this context. Indeed, MI cannot be ruled out with 100% certainty in the time period during which fibrinolytic therapy is most effective.

As outlined above, in Western Europe and the United States pre-hospital initiation of fibrinolytic treatment reduces the call-to-needle time by about 1 hour compared to in-hospital therapy. The gain of earlier therapy is

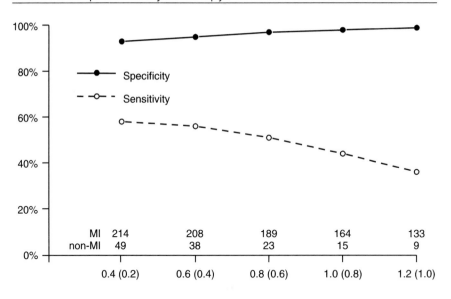

Figure 7.7

Sensitivity and specificity in confirmation of myocardial infarction at several thresholds of ST deviation on the presenting ECGs. All 263 (214+49) patients in this figure met the classical criteria for in-hospital confirmation of infarction (≥2 leads of VI–V6 show ≥0.2 mV ST elevation or ≥2 leads of II,III,aVF show ≥0.1 mV ST elevation). ST deviation is defined as: (a) in case of anterior ST elevation: the total sum of ST elevation in V1–V6 plus ST depression in II,III,aVF; and (b) otherwise (said to be inferior): the total sum of ST elevation in I,II,III,aVF,aVL,V5,V6 plus ST depression in V1–V4. Adapted from Boersma et al (1998).[25]

time-dependent (Figs 7.3 and 7.4). The average gain per hour earlier treatment is approximately 60, 10 and 2 lives saved per 1000 treated patients in the respective 0–1 hour, >1–3 hour and >3–6 hour intervals after onset of symptoms. If pre-hospital fibrinolysis were restricted to patients presenting within 6 hours, on average, mortality reduction in definite MI patients—the *benefit* of a pre-hospital fibrinolysis programme—can reliably be estimated at 10–20 lives saved per 1000 treated. In some patients, an intracranial bleeding may occur as a consequence of fibrinolytic therapy, which will lead to death in more than half of the cases and to severe disability in another quarter.[26] The risk for intracranial haemorrhage (ICH) can be estimated at 5–10 per 1000 patients treated.[9,26] In patients with evolving MI this risk is partly compensated by a reduction of the risk for embolic stroke (strokes of any type occur in approximately 4–8 per 1000 treated patients).[9,26] Moreover, the expected mortality reduction far exceeds the expected risk of ICH.[9] However, in patients without infarction who (erroneously) receive fibrinolytic therapy the benefits are absent, while the bleeding risk prevails. Hence, the *risk* of a pre-hospital fibrinolysis programme can be estimated at 5–10 intracranial bleeding complications per 1000 treated non-infarctions. Figure 7.8 presents the expected benefit/risk ratio at several thresholds of ST deviation. In the above-mentioned series of 1072 patients, for each 4 patients with a confirmed infarction who met the classical ST thresholds 1 patient without confirmed infarction did so, resulting in a benefit/risk ratio of 4–17.[25] This ratio can be improved by introducing additional criteria for total ST deviation, or by using more strict criteria for ST elevation. Although the question of the optimal ratio between benefits and risks in pre-hospital fibrinolysis cannot be answered unambiguously, these data may be of help to make rational choices in clinical practice. It should be realized in this respect that a relatively high benefit/risk ratio will result in a relatively high net benefit (estimated benefit minus risk; interpretation: the additional number of lives saved by pre-hospital treatment without additional cerebral complications) per patient *treated*, but in a relatively low net benefit per patient *screened*.

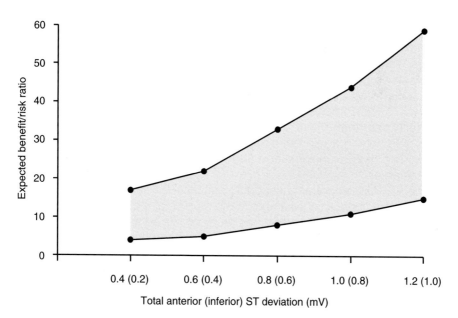

Figure 7.8

Expected benefit/risk ratio at several thresholds of ST deviation on the presenting ECGs. Only the 263 patients that met the classical in-hospital criteria (Fig. 7.7) for confirmation of infarction are potential candidates for pre-hospital fibrinolysis. These patients contribute in the benefit/risk estimations. See Fig. 7.7 for the definition of ST deviation. Adapted from Boersma et al (1998).[25]

Pre-hospital fibrinolysis: the Dutch experience

In 1988 a programme for pre-hospital triage and fibrinolytic treatment was initiated in the Rotterdam area of The Netherlands.[27–29] Table 7.3 shows the *in-* and *ex*clusion criteria for eligibility of pre-hospital fibrinolysis according to this REPerfusion in Acute Infarction Rotterdam (REPAIR) programme. In case of a suspected AMI the general practitioner, or, in his absence, the ambulance nurse applies a short questionnaire. A portable device equipped with a computer algorithm acquires a standard 12-lead simultaneous ECG. If the device detects a major evolving MI and the questionnaire confirms patient eligibility, the ambulance nurse initiates fibrinolytic therapy, and the crew will transport the patient to the hospital.

From June 1988 to June 2000 a total of 1487 patients have received fibrinolytic treatment according to the REPAIR protocol. Of all patients 56%, 80% and 90% notified the emergency service within 1, 2 and 3 hours, respectively. In 9 patients (0.6%) pre-hospital fibrinolytic treatment was initiated whereas the diagnosed MI could not be confirmed during hospital admission. One of these patients suffered a non-fatal haemorrhagic stroke. Two patients died during transportation, whereas ventricular fibrillation occurred in 40 patients (2.7%), all of whom were successfully resuscitated. No major haemorrhagic complications occurred during transportation. Mortality after 30 days, 1, 5 and 10 years was 4.9%, 7.3%, 16.2%, and 30.1%, respectively. These results are highly motivating: note that 30 day and 1 year survival in recent clinical trials of MI patients are in the range 5.5–7% and 9–11%, respectively.[17,18,30–33] Patients treated within 2 hours had a significantly lower mortality rate than those treated within 2–6 hours from symptom onset (Fig. 7.9), which again emphasized the importance of very early treatment. The difference remained after adjustment for age and other clinical variables.

The REPAIR programme set out to evaluate the safety and feasibility of pre-hospital fibrinolytic treatment in the municipal area of Rotterdam. The positive outcome of this project has prompted its continuation and integration into routine care of the Rotterdam ambulance emergency service. To date, approximately 10% of myocardial infarction patients in the region of Rotterdam receive fibrinolytic therapy before hospital admission according to the REPAIR protocol.

Another aspect of very early lysis of the intracoronary thrombus is that the infarct process can be aborted in a stage at which irreversible myocardial damage has not yet occurred. Lamfers et al. defined an aborted infarction by fibrinolytic treatment as follows: (1) a patient has chest pain and ECG changes suggestive of transmural ischaemia; (2) the cumulative sum of ST-segment elevation and depression decreased to <50% within 2 hours of treatment; and (3) creatine kinase myoglobin

Table 7.3 Main *in-* and *exclusion* criteria for pre-hospital fibrinolytic treatment according to the REPAIR programme.

Inclusion criteria

1988 Initial
- chest pain suggestive of myocardial infarction, existing ≤3 hours
- pain not responsive to nitroglycerin
- upper age limit 70 years; for women: lower age limit 55 years (to exclude potential pregnancy)

1991 Modification
- chest pain suggestive of myocardial infarction, existing ≤6 hours
- upper age limit 75 years; lower age limit for women dropped, but pregnancy remains an exclusion criteria

1996 Modification
- upper age limit 80 years

Exclusion criteria

1988 Initial
- cardiopulmonary resuscitation
- history of stroke
- severe trauma
- lowered conciousness
- uncontrolled hypertension
- recent history of blood loss
- paresis or paralysis
- use of oral anticoagulants
- surgery within past 3 months
- hypersensitivity to streptokinase

1991 Modification
- pregnancy
- use of oral anticoagulants allowed

Electrocardiographic criteria

1988 Initial
- ≥3 mm ST elevation in ≥2 precordial leads OR ≥2 mm ST elevation in ≥2 limb leads
- total sum of ST deviation ≥10 mm

1996 Modification
- ≥2 mm ST elevation in ≥2 precordial leads AND ≥3 mm ST elevation in ≥1 precordial leads
- total sum of ST deviation ≥6 (8) mm in case of age ≤70 (80) years
OR
- ≥1 mm ST elevation in ≥2 limb leads AND ≥2 mm ST elevation in ≥1 limb leads
- total sum of ST deviation ≥4 (6) mm in case of age ≤70 (80) years

2001 Modification
- total sum of ST deviation ≥15 mm: eligible for primary percutaneous coronary intervention (PCI)

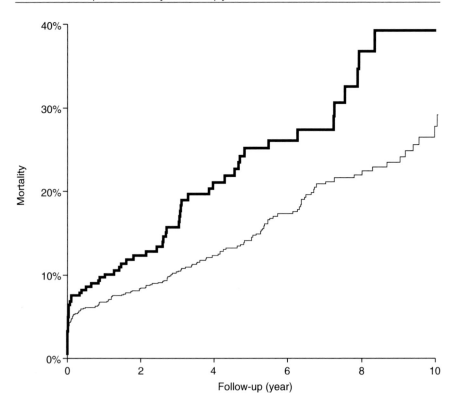

Figure 7.9

Long-term follow-up of the 1487 patients treated according to the REPAIR protocol.
The thin line represents patients treated within 2 hours from onset of symptoms; the bold
line represents patients treated between 2 hours and 6 hours. Adapted from Boersma et al
(2001).[29]

fraction (CK-MB) elevations remained below 2 times the upper limit of
normal.[34] In a series of 224 MI patients who were treated before hospital
admission according to the Nijmegen pre-hospital treatment programme
13% fulfilled these criteria, as compared to 4% in a comparable series of
266 patients who received in-hospital treatment.[34] Thus, pre-hospital fibrinolysis is associated with a higher (order of magnitude: 3-fold) proportion
of patients with aborted infarction than in-hospital treatment. The need to
start treatment before hospital admission is sometimes questioned by
cardiologists who argue that transportation times in their region are short,
whereas, in their practice, fibrinolytic therapy will be applied very early
after hospital arrival. At this time, we waive the fact that physicians tend to
have an optimistic view on their own practices (see the registries data
presented above). Here is the ultimate litmus-test proof to this
critical assertion: just count the number of aborted infarctions in your
practice.

Fibrinolysis or primary angioplasty?

Timing of coronary blood flow restoration is important, but is not the sole determinant of the end result. Additional factors are TIMI flow and the occurrence of coronary reocclusion. Recent studies have shown that fibrinolytic treatment is capable of restoring coronary patency in 55–80% of cases, depending on the fibrinolytic agent used.[35] Thus, coronary reperfusion does not occur in 20–45% of patients. In addition, 5–10% of patients experience an early reocclusion, whereas 30% experience late occlusion.[36,37] An alternative approach to reopen the occluded coronary vessel is to perform a percutaneous coronary intervention (PCI), which is known to have a success rate of 95–99%.[38] The most prominent disadvantage of this approach is the inherent treatment delay involved in mobilizing the interventional team and readying the interventional facility. Under optimal circumstances, this will lead to a—costly—30 min treatment delay as compared with in-hospital initiation of fibrinolytic therapy. When compared to pre-hospital treatment, this delay will amount to 60–90 min. Randomized trials have shown an additional survival benefit for PCI when compared to *in*-hosptial fibrinolytic treatment.[38] To date, there are no large-scale data available on direct comparisons of PCI and *pre*-hospital fibrinolytic treatment. The small CAPTIM trial hints at an equal outcome when using either treatment modality.[39] Results of indirect comparisons lead to a similar conclusion. The meta-analysis of randomized trials of PCI versus fibrinolysis reported an absolute 30 day mortality reduction of 2.1%, and a proportional mortality reduction of 34% (95% CI 6–54%).[38] The meta-analysis of randomized trials of pre-hospital versus in-hospital treatment demonstrate a 1.7% absolute mortality reduction (or 20/1000 treated patients per 1 hour earlier treatment, Fig. 7.6), and an 18% proportional reduction (95% CI 3–30%).[40] The 5 year mortality reduction by primary angioplasty in the Zwolle study (absolute 10.5%; proportional 46% and 95% CI 13–64%) is similar to the 5 year mortality reduction by pre-hospital fibrinolysis in GREAT (absolute 10.6%; proportional 30% and 95% CI: 2–63%).[41,42]

In view of these data, both strategies should not be considered competitors, but as complementary parts of an umbrella reperfusion strategy. Such a strategy should aim at a rapid and accurate diagnosis, and—after MI is confirmed—reperfusion therapy tailored to the clinical presentation of the individual patient and the locally available facilities. The location and the extent of the jeopardized myocardium, the risk of bleeding complications and the time from onset of symptoms to treatment will play key roles in this respect.[43] Primary angioplasty should be considered the treatment of choice in well-equipped and experienced centres. The vast majority of patients, however, have no access to these facilities, and will benefit more from immediate fibrinolytic treatment. To date, sophisticated portable electrocardiographic devices and easy to use fibrinolytic agents (bolus injections) are available to facilitate such home diagnosis and home treatment.

References

1. Herrick JB. Clinical features of sudden obstruction of the coronary arteries. JAMA 1912; **59**:2015.

2. DeWood MA, Spores J, Notske R et al. Prevalence of total coronary artery occlusion during the early hours of transmural myocardial infarction. N Engl J Med 1980; **303**:897–902.

3. Flameng W, Lesaffre E, Vanhaecke J. Determinants of infarct size in non-human primates. Bas Res Cardiol 1990; **85**:392–403.

4. Reimer KA, Heide van der RS, Richard VJ. Reperfusion in acute myocardial infarction: effect of timing and modulating factors in experimental models. Am J Cardiol 1993; **72**(suppl):13G–21G.

5. Reimer KA, Lowe JE, Rasmussen MM, Jennings RB. The wavefront phenomenon of ischemic cell death: 1. Myocardial infarct size versus duration of coronary occlusion in dogs. Circulation 1977; **56**:786–94.

6. Dorado DG, Théroux P, Elizaga J et al. Myocardial infarction in the pig heart model: infarct size and duration of coronary occlusion. Cardiovasc Res 1987; **21**: 537–44.

7. Schaper W, Binz K, Sass S, Winkler B. Influence of collateral blood flow and of variations in MVO_2 on tissue-ATP content in ischemic and infarcted myocardium. J Mol Cell Cardiol 1987; **19**:19–37.

8. Hermens WT, Willems GM, Nijssen KM, Simoons ML. Effect of thrombolytic treatment delay on myocardial infarction size. Lancet 1992; **340**:1297 (Letter to the editor).

9. Fibrinolytic Therapy Trialists' (FTT) Collaborative Group. Indications for fibrinolytic therapy in suspected acute myocardial infarction: collaborative overview of early mortality and major morbidity results from all randomised trials of more than 1,000 patients. Lancet 1994; **343**: 311–22.

10. Boersma E, Maas ACP, Deckers JW, Simoons ML. Early thrombolytic treatment in acute myocardial infarction: reappraisal of the golden hour. Lancet 1996; **348**:771–5.

11. Weaver WD. Time to thrombolytic treatment: factors affecting delay and their influence on outcome. J Am Coll Cardiol 1995; **25**(suppl):3S–9S.

12. Hasdai D, Behar S, Wallentin L et al. A prospective survey of the characteristics, treatments and outcomes of patients with acute coronary syndromes in Europe and the Mediterranean Basin: The Euro Heart Survey of Acute Coronary Syndromes. Eur Heart J 2002; **23**:1190–201.

13. European Myocardial Infarction Project Group. Prehospital thrombolytic therapy in patients with suspected acute myocardial infarction. N Engl J Med 1993; **329**:383–9.

14. Weaver WD, Cerqueira M, Hallstrom AP et al. for the Myocardial Infarction Triage and Intervention Project Group. Prehospital-initiated vs

hospital-initiated thrombolytic therapy. The Myocardial Infarction Triage and Intervention trial. JAMA 1993; **270**:1211–16.

15. GREAT Group. Feasibility, safety, and efficacy of domiciliary thrombolysis by general practitioners: Grampian Region Early Anistreplase Trial. BMJ 1992; **305**:548–53.

16. Task Force on the management of acute myocardial infarction of the European Society of Cardiology. Acute myocardial infarction: prehospital and inhospital management. Eur Heart J 1996; **17**:43–63.

17. GUSTO investigators. An international randomized trial comparing four thrombolytic strategies for acute myocardial infarction. N Engl J Med 1993; **329**: 673–82.

18. White H. Thrombin-specific anticoagulation with bivalirudin versus heparin in patients receiving fibrinolytic therapy for acute myocardial infarction: the HERO-2 randomised trial. Lancet 2001; **358**:1855–63.

19. McNeill AJ, Cunningham SR, Flannery DJ et al. A double blind placebo controlled study of early and late administration of recombinant tissue plasminogen activator in acute myocardial infarction. Br Heart J 1989; **61**:316–21.

20. Schofer J, Büttner J, Geng G et al. Prehospital thrombolysis in acute myocardial infarction. Am J Cardiol 1990; **66**:1429–33.

21. Barbash GI, Roth A, Hod H et al. Improved survival but not left ventricular function with early and prehospital treatment with tissue plasminogen activator in acute myocardial infarction. Am J Cardiol 1990; **66**:261–6.

22. Castaigne AD, Hervé C, Duval-Moulin AM et al. Pre-hospital use of APSAC: results of a placebo-controlled study. Am J Cardiol 1989; **64**(suppl):30A–33A.

23. McAleer B, Ruane B, Burke E et al. Prehospital thrombolysis in a rural cummunity: short- and long-term survival. Cardiovasc Drugs Ther 1992; **6**:369–72.

24. Adams J, Trent R, Rawles J on behalf of the GREAT Group. Earliest electrocardiographic evidence of myocardial infarction: implications for thrombolytic treatment. BMJ 1993; **307**: 409–13.

25. Boersma H, Maas ACP, Grijseels EWM, Deckers JW, Harman JAM, Simoons ML. Benefits and risks of possible prehospital thrombolysis strategies—the role of the electrocardiogram. Cardiologie 1998; **5**: 562–8.

26. Gore JM, Granger CB, Simoons ML et al. for the GUSTO-1 investigators. Stroke after thrombolysis: mortality and functional outcomes in the GUSTO-1 trial. Circulation 1995; **92**:2811–18.

27. Bouten MJM, Simoons ML, Hartman JAM, Van Miltenburg AJM, Van der Does E, Pool J. Prehospital thrombolysis with alteplase (rt-PA) in acute myocardial infarction. Eur Heart J 1992; **13**:925–31.

28. Grijseels EW, Bouten MJ, Lenderink T et al. Pre-hospital thrombolytic therapy with either alteplase or streptokinase. Practical applications, complications and long-term results in 529 patients. Eur Heart J 1995; **16**:1833–8.

29. Boersma E, Maas ACP, Harman JAM, Ilmer B, Vos J, Simoons ML. 12 jaar triage en trombolytische behandelin voor ziekenhuisopname bij hartinfarctpatienten in de regio Rotterdam: uitstekende korte- en langetermijnresultaten [Summary

in English]. Ned Tijdschr Geneesk 2001; **145**:2029–35.

30. GUSTO-3 investigators. A comparison of reteplase with alteplase for acute myocardial infarction. N Engl J Med 1997; **337**:1118–23.

31. ASSENT-2 investigators. Single-bolus tenecteplase compared with front-loaded alteplase in acute myocardial infarction: the ASSENT-2 double-blind randomised trial. Assessment of the Safety and Efficacy of a New Thrombolytic Investigators. Lancet 1999; **354**:716–22.

32. Topol EJ. Reperfusion therapy for acute myocardial infarction with fibrinolytic therapy or combination reduced fibrinolytic therapy and platelet glycoprotein IIb/IIIa inhibition: the GUSTO V randomised trial. Lancet 2001; **357**:1905–14.

33. ASSENT-3 investigators. Efficacy and safety of tenecteplase in combination with enoxaparin, abciximab, or unfractionated heparin: the ASSENT-3 randomised trial in acute myocardial infarction. Lancet 2001; **358**:605–13.

34. Lamfers EJP, Hooghoudt TEH, Uppelschoten A, Stolwijk PWJ, Verheugt FWA. Effect of prehospital thrombolysis on aborting acute myocardial infarction. Am J Cardiol 1999; **84**:928–30.

35. Grines CL. Should thrombolysis or primary angioplasty be the treatment of choice for acute myocardial infarction? Primary angioplasty—the strategy of choice. N Engl J Med 1996; **335**:1313–16.

36. Meijer A, Verheugt FW, Werter CJ, Lie KI, Van der Pol JM, Van Eenige MJ. Aspirin versus coumadin in the prevention of reocclusion and recurrent ischemia after successful thrombolysis: a prospective placebo-controlled angiographic study. Results of the APRICOT Study. Circulation 1993; **87**:1524–30.

37. GUSTO Angiographic Investigators.The effects of tissue plasminogen activator, streptokinase, or both on coronary-artery patency, ventricular function, and survival after acute myocardial infarction. N Engl J Med 1993; **329**:1615–22.

38. Weaver WD, Simes RJ, Betriu A et al. Comparison of primary coronary angioplasty and intravenous thrombolytic therapy for acute myocardial infarction: a quantitative review. JAMA 1997; **278**:2093–8.

39. Bonnefoy E, Lapostolle F, Leizorovicz A et al. Primary angioplasty versus prehospital fibrinolysis in acute myocardial infarction: a randomised study. Lancet 2002; **360**:825–9.

40. Boersma E, Akkerhuis KM, Simoons ML. Primary angioplasty versus thrombolysis for acute myocardial infarction. N Engl J Med 2000; **342**:890–1 (Letter).

41. Zijlstra F, Hoorntje JCA, De Boer MJ et al. Long-term benefit of primary angioplasty as compared with thrombolytic therapy for acute myocardial infarction. N Engl J Med 1999; **341**:1413–19.

42. Rawles JM. Quantification of the benefit of earlier thrombolytic therapy: five-year results of the Grampian Region Early Anistreplase Trial (GREAT). J Am Coll Cardiol 1997; **30**:1181–6.

43. Boersma E, Van der Vlugt MJ, Steyerberg EW, Simoons ML. Reperfusion therapy for acute myocardial infarction. Which strategy for which patient? Drugs 1998; **56**:31–48.

8
Fibrinolytic therapy in venous thromboembolism

Marije ten Wolde, Maria M W Koopman and Harry R Büller

Introduction

Acute venous thromboembolism includes deep vein thrombosis of the leg and pulmonary embolism. It is a frequently occurring disease with a potentially fatal outcome. The clinical course is characterized by short-term as well as long-term sequelae. The main goal for therapy, therefore, is to prevent extension and recurrence of the disease in the acute phase and to prevent long-term complications, such as the post-thrombotic syndrome and pulmonary hypertension.

Although deep vein thrombosis and pulmonary embolism traditionally are defined as two different clinical entities, they are now more seen as manifestations of one and the same disease, venous thromboembolism. Venographic studies in patients with pulmonary embolism revealed that around 80% of them have evidence of thrombosis in the leg.[1,2] Vice versa, in 50–80% of patients with deep vein thrombosis, silent pulmonary embolism is present as revealed by ventilation perfusion scintigraphy.[3] However, most of the available treatment studies were designed and executed separately for the two diseases. In this chapter, therefore, first the epidemiology, natural history and prognosis of deep vein thrombosis will be briefly discussed followed by a review of the anticoagulant and fibrinolytic therapy for this disease. Subsequently, the same issues regarding pulmonary embolism will be discussed and finally some recommendations will be made.

Deep vein thrombosis (DVT)

Background: epidemiology, natural history and prognosis

Deep vein thrombosis of the leg is a common disease with an annual incidence of 1–2 per 1000 individuals per year.[4] The acute symptoms consist of redness, swelling and pain due to venous obstruction and inflammation. Later sequelae include recurrent DVT or pulmonary embolism and the post-thrombotic syndrome. Follow-up studies of patients with a first episode of thrombosis showed that the cumulative risk for recurrent disease is about 30% over 8 years and that approximately 50% of patients will develop the post-thrombotic syndrome in the subsequent 2 years following the thrombotic event.[5] The main goal of therapy, therefore, is to prevent extension or recurrence of the disease and to impede the late effects of venous thrombosis. To achieve this goal, different therapeutic approaches are available, such as thrombectomy, fibrinolytic therapy and treatment with anticoagulant drugs. The most accepted treatment for deep vein thrombosis is anticoagulant therapy.

Anticoagulant therapy: heparin and vitamin K antagonists

It is current practice to treat patients with proven acute deep vein thrombosis (DVT) initially with heparin or low molecular weight heparin (LMWH) for a period of 5–7 days, followed by vitamin K antagonists for at least 3 months. At least 14 well-designed studies have compared the treatment of activated partial thromboplastin time (APTT) adjusted heparin with fixed-dose LMWH in the initial phase of DVT treatment. During a 3–6 months follow-up period, 4.3% of the patients treated with LMWH experienced recurrent thrombotic events as compared to 5.6% in the patients who received unfractionated heparin (OR 0.76; 95% CI 0.57–1.01).[6] Major bleeding occurred in 1.3% of the patients in the LMWH group and in 2.1% of the patients treated with standard unfractionated heparin (OR 0.60; 95% CI: 0.39–0.93). Hence, the current therapy of LMWH and vitamin K antagonists is very effective in preventing recurrent disease with a low risk of bleeding. It is, however, unknown what the efficacy is in preventing the post-thrombotic syndrome. The etiology of the post-thrombotic syndrome is thought to be caused by venous valve damage, regurgitation of blood, venous hypertension and stenosis.[7] Early clot lysis could be an attractive option to prevent valve damage, persistent stenosis and in the end venous hypertension. Therefore, fibrinolytic therapy may be useful.

Fibrinolytic therapy

Recently, Wells and Forster reviewed the available literature regarding fibrinolytics in the treatment of DVT.[8] A total of seven randomized trials have compared treatment of streptokinase with unfractionated heparin (UFH) in the treatment of patients with proximal DVT. Streptokinase was administered as a bolus injection (range 50 000–600 000 U) followed by continuous infusion (100 000–200 000 U/hour) over a time period ranging from 1 to 7 days. Outcome measures were short-term efficacy, adverse events and incidence of the post-thrombotic syndrome. Short-term efficacy was evaluated by comparing pre- and post-treatment venograms. A good response was defined differently in the various studies and included moderate to substantial clot lysis, > 50% lysis or grade III–IV lysis. Adverse events were defined as major bleeding, or death. The presence of the post-thrombotic syndrome was assessed clinically with knowledge of treatment allocation and in all studies patients were lost to follow-up; hence these data are likely to be biased. Table 8.1 shows the short-term efficacy results and bleeding rates of the seven studies.[9–15] It is clear from this table that the administration of streptokinase is associated with a 4-fold greater significant clot lysis at the cost of a 3-fold increase in bleeding. The rate of major haemorrhages was 15% in streptokinase-treated patients as compared to 5% in heparin recipients. Three other studies have compared rt-PA (alteplase) and UFH with placebo and UFH in patients with proximal DVT.[16–18] In one study rt-PA was given as a bolus (range 0.5 mg/kg over 4 hours–0.5 mg/kg over 8 hours) and repeated after 24 h; in another study, rt-PA was administered as a continuous infusion (0.05 mg/kg/h over 1 day); whereas, in the third study, patients received a continuous infusion of 100 mg on day 1, followed by a continuous infusion of 50 mg on the second day. Outcome events were venographic clot lysis, major haemorrhage and pulmonary embolism. In Table 8.2, the results with respect to efficacy (>50% clot lysis) and safety of these three studies are summarized. Again, there is a significant increase of clot lysis in those patients receiving fibrinolytic therapy (RR 8.1; 95% CI 2.2–29.6), which is accompanied by an (insignificant) increased risk of major bleeding (RR 1.6; 95% CI 0.4–6.4). Pulmonary embolism was not observed in these studies. Finally, there are two trials comparing urokinase with UFH.[19,20] In the first study, 250 000 U urokinase as a bolus was administered followed by 750 000 U over 25 min, while in the other study 200 000 U urokinase over 24 hours was given. Based on a total of 37 patients, these studies showed nonsignificant differences in venographic efficacy and safety.

Taken together, the results of all studies show a similar picture in that early efficacy in terms of vein patency is better in patients treated with fibrinolytics as compared to unfractionated heparin. However, it remains unproven that this better venographic vein patency rate results in a lower risk of the post-thrombotic syndrome. Moreover, the price to be paid is a much higher risk for major bleeding. Therefore, fibrinolytic therapy for DVT should not be applied unless in the setting of a clinical study to assess the real value in the prevention of the post-thrombotic syndrome.

Catheter-directed fibrinolytic therapy
Catheter-directed fibrinolytic therapy involves administration of the fibrinolytic agent directly at the site of the thrombus using a catheter. Many access routes have been used, such as the internal jugular vein, contralateral femoral vein as well as the ipsilateral femoral or popliteal

Table 8.1 The efficacy (as assessed by repeat venography) and safety of streptokinase vs heparin for the initial treatment of acute deep vein thrombosis.

Study	No. of patients	Treatment groups		Significant lysis		Major haemorrhage	
		T(+H)	H	T(+H)	H	T(+H)	H
Robertson et al (1968)[10]	16	Streptokinase + heparin	Heparin	5/8	1/8	2/8	0/8
Kakkar et al (1969)[11]	20	Streptokinase	Heparin	7/10	2/10	3/10	2/10
Robertson et al (1970)[9]	16	Streptokinase + heparin	Heparin	5/9	1/7	1/9	0/7
Tsapogas et al (1973)[12]	34	Streptokinase + heparin	Heparin	10/19	1/15	4/19	0/15
Porter et al (1975)[15]	50	Streptokinase + heparin	Heparin	13/24	8/26	4/24	1/26
Elliot et al (1979)[13]	51	Streptokinase + heparin	Heparin	17/26	0/25	2/26	0/25
Arnesen et al (1978)[14]	42	Streptokinase	Heparin	15/21	5/21	2/21	2/21
Total	229	Streptokinase + heparin	Heparin	72/117 (62%)	18/112 (16%)	18/117 (15%)	5/112 (5%)
Relative risk (95% CI)				3.9 (2.5–6.0) Test for heterogeneity $p = 0.21$		2.8 (1.2–6.2) Test for heterogeneity $p = 0.85$	

T, thrombolysis; H, heparin.

Table 8.2 The efficacy (as assessed by repeat venography) and safety of rt-PA vs heparin for the initial treatment of acute deep vein thrombosis

Study	No. of patients	Treatment groups		Significant lysis		Major haemorrhage	
		T(+H)	H	T(+H)	H	T(+H)	H
Verhaeghe et al (1989)[18]	32	rt-PA + heparin	Heparin	na	na	8/25	0/7
Goldhaber et al (1990)[17]	65	rt-PA (N = 36) rt-PA + heparin (N = 17)	Heparin Heparin	15/53	0/12	1/53	0/12
Turpie et al (1990)[16]	83	rt-PA + heparin	Heparin	13/41	2/42	1/41	2/42
Total	148	rt-PA	Heparin	28/94 (30%)	2/54 (4%)	10/119 (8%)	2/61 (3%)
Relative risk (95% CI)				8.1 (2.2–29.6) Test for heterogeneity p = 0.7		1.6 (0.4–6.4) Test for heterogeneity p = 0.4	

na, not available because percentage clot lysis is not reported; T, thrombolysis; H, heparin.

vein. Initially, urokinase has been used and more recently rt-PA. There are no randomized trials comparing catheter-directed fibrinolytic therapy with standard anticoagulant therapy for deep vein thrombosis. Recently, a review describing several case reports and case series has been published.[21] In this review 263 patients were treated with catheter-directed fibrinolytics for ileofemoral or caval vein thrombosis. A total of 221 (84%) of the patients had a good short-term outcome in terms of vein patency and 4.9% suffered from major bleeding. Long-term outcome was not reported. Also, the results of an American multi-centre registry of patients treated with catheter-directed fibrinolytic therapy has recently been published.[22] In this registry, data of 473 patients treated with catheter-directed fibrinolytics were recorded. After 1 week only 287 (61%) patients could be analysed. Venous patency rates were 83% in the first week, but after 6 months 65% and after 12 months 60%. This is comparable with the standard treatment with low molecular weight heparins (LMWHs) and vitamin K antagonists. Major bleeding occurred in 16% of the patients and 0.4% of the patients died as a direct result of the fibrinolytic therapy. Therefore, based on these data, the role for catheter-directed fibrinolytic therapy is limited and the benefits are unproven. Possibly the only exception is a severe clinical presentation of deep vein thrombosis, such as phlegmasia coerulea dolens.

Pulmonary embolism

Background: epidemiology, natural history and prognosis

Pulmonary embolism (PE) involves an occlusion of one or more pulmonary arteries by material originating from outside the pulmonary circulation, usually the deep leg veins. Symptoms of PE include shortness of breath, pleuritic chest pain, haemoptysis, and sometimes syncope. These symptoms are not specific; after objective testing with imaging techniques, such as ventilation perfusion scintigraphy and pulmonary angiography, the disease is confirmed in only 20–30% of patients presenting with a suspicion of PE. Pulmonary embolism is a relatively frequently occurring disease: the estimated annual incidence is about 1–2 per 1000 inhabitants in the Western world.[23,24] However, it is difficult to estimate the real incidence of PE since many cases are unrecognized, as revealed by autopsy studies.[25]

Based on reports from the mid-twentieth century, the mortality rate of untreated PE seems to vary around 25%.[26–28] It has to be noted that at that time the diagnosis was based on a combination of symptoms and signs and information from chest X-ray and electrocardiogram. Since Barrit and Jordan reported their landmark randomized controlled trial in 1960 of anticoagulants (a combination of vitamin K antagonists and heparin) versus no treatment, anticoagulant therapy has become standard in the management of PE.[28] The trial stopped prematurely after 35 patients had been included because in the 19 untreated patients, 5 died of PE and 5 other patients developed non-fatal recurrences, whereas in the 16 treated patients only 1 patient died due to another reason. Although survival has improved considerably with adequate anticoagulant treatment, the PE-related mortality rates in the first 3–6 months remain 3–8%.[29-31] Hence, there is a need for more effective therapeutic modalities.

Anticoagulant treatment: heparin and vitamin K antagonists

Standard anticoagulant therapy for patients with acute PE consists of unfractionated heparin (UFH) followed by vitamin K antagonists. UFH is given by intravenous pump infusion for at least 5 days in a dose that is adjusted to prolong the activated partial thromboplastin time 1.5–2.5 times the normal range.[32,33] Vitamin K antagonists are started with UFH and can be discontinued when the international normalized ratio (INR) is in the therapeutic range 2.0–3.0 for 2 consecutive days. Patients with a first episode of PE should be treated for at least 3 months.[34] The principal aims of this treatment are to prevent thrombus extension and the occurrence of new pulmonary emboli with a minimal risk of bleeding. Two large clinical studies have shown that low molecular weight heparins (LMWHs) are as effective and safe as UFH for the initial treatment of pulmonary embolism. Because the total amount of patients studied is much smaller as compared to that for the treatment of DVT,[35] UFH remains the standard therapy for patients with acute PE, although LMWH is a good alternative.

Fibrinolytic therapy

Fibrinolytic therapy has been investigated as the initial treatment in patients with acute PE for many years. The rationale for the use of fibrinolytic therapy is based on the expected more rapid thrombus resolution compared to heparin therapy alone. As a result, lung perfusion will be restored more quickly with a potential clinical benefit. Moreover, right ventricular overload could be decreased which might prevent right ventricular failure, systemic hypotension, shock and ultimately death. Also long-term clinical benefit could theoretically be achieved by preventing chronic right ventricular dysfunction and pulmonary hypertension. Last, recurrences of PE could be prevented because of the more complete resolution of the source of emboli.

Efficacy of fibrinolytic therapy: surrogate markers
The theory that pulmonary perfusion will be more rapidly restored by fibrinolytic therapy ('thrombolysis') is supported by several clinical

reports. In a study with 36 selected patients treated with rt-PA, 34 of the 36 patients showed thrombus resolution as assessed by follow-up angiography after 2–6 hours.[36] Comparison with heparin is possible in the randomized controlled UPET,[37] PIOPED[38] and PAIMS-2[39] trials, which showed more thrombus resolution 2 hours after thrombolysis as compared to heparin therapy. Table 8.3 summarizes the effects in the different studies of thrombolysis as compared to heparin alone with respect to scintigraphic thrombus resolution. After 24 hours significant differences in thrombus resolution exist in favour of thrombolysis. However, when lung perfusion is compared in a later stage—i.e. after 7 days,[38,40,41] 30 days,[39] and 1 year[37]—these differences are no longer detectable.

When right ventricular function is considered as an outcome measure for the efficacy of fibrinolytic treatment the same pattern is observed. Short-term improvement of right ventricular function is achieved in patients receiving fibrinolytic treatment. In a study with 7 patients receiving rt-PA, right ventricular wall movement normalized in 5 patients and improved in 2.[42] In a non-randomized prospective trial of 40 patients with major PE receiving heparin (13 patients) or rt-PA (27 patients), signs of echocardiographic right ventricular overload (such as right ventricular dilatation, paradoxal septal movement, inspiratory collapse of the vena cava) were significantly less after 12 hours in the group treated with rt-PA, as compared to heparin recipients.[43] One randomized trial evaluated right ventricular function in patients who received either rt-PA or heparin.[40] After 3 hours, improvement of right ventricular wall motion occurred in 29% of patients receiving rt-PA, whereas it improved in 13% of the heparin recipients. After 24 hours these figures were 39% and 17%, respectively. However, in the study of Konstantinides et al the signs of acute right ventricular pressure overload progressively resolved at follow-up echocardiography after 48 hours and 7 days, regardless of the type of treatment.[43]

Taken together, these results suggest that thrombolysis induces early reperfusion of lung tissue and improvement of right ventricular function, an effect that can also be attained by heparin alone, albeit at a slower pace.

Efficacy of fibrinolytic therapy: clinical outcomes

How do these findings on surrogate markers translate into clinical outcomes? The largest clinical trial of thrombolysis versus heparin is the UPET trial, reported in 1970.[37] In this trial, 82 patients were randomized to urokinase followed by heparin, whereas the other 78 patients received heparin alone. In the urokinase group, 6 patients developed a PE recurrence (of which 1 episode was fatal) and 6 patients died. In the heparin group, 5 patients had a PE recurrence and 7 patients died. Thus, no clear differences were observed between the two treatment groups in clinical

Table 8.3 Scintigraphic thrombus resolution after thrombolysis and heparin as compared to heparin alone.

Study	Treatment regimens		Lung scintigraphic thrombus resolution (relative difference in not perfused lung proportion)					
			t = 24 hours		t = 5–7days		t = 30–90 days	
	T+H	H	T+H	H	T+H	H	T+H	H
UPET (1970)[37]	Urokinase 4400 U/kg + 4400 U/kg/h for 12 hours + heparin (N = 72)	Heparin (N = 70)	22%	8%	41% (N = 67)	36%[a] (N = 59)	71% (N = 29)	73%[a] (N = 28)
Levine et al (1990)[41]	rt-PA 0.6 mg/kg/2 min + heparin (N = 33)	Heparin (N = 25)	37%	19%	58%	49%[a]	na	na
PIOPED (1990)[38]	40–80 mg/40–90 min rt-PA + heparin (N = 9)	Heparin (N = 4)	26%	0%[a]	51%	17%[a]	na	na
PAIMS-2 (1992)[39]	100 mg/2 h rt-PA + heparin (N = 20)	Heparin (N = 16)	na	na	41%	37%[a]	54%	68%[a]
Goldhaber et al (1993)[40]	100 mg/2 hours rt-PA + heparin (N = 46)	Heparin (N = 55)	34%	4%	na	na	na	na

[a] Differences not statistically significant; T, thrombolysis; H, heparin.

outcome. Since 1990, several randomized trials comparing the fibrinolytic agent rt-PA to heparin alone have been conducted using different dosing regimens. The findings of these studies are detailed in Table 8.4. No significant differences in venous thromboembolism (VTE) recurrences and mortality could be observed, although the sample sizes of the individual studies were small. Patients treated with heparin have a 1.3 times higher risk regarding all-cause mortality than patients receiving thrombolysis; however, this result is not statistically significant. Although neither are statistically significant, there appears to be a beneficial effect of thrombolysis as compared to heparin with respect to PE-related mortality and VTE recurrences (RR 1.6; 95% CI 0.5–5.3 and RR 1.4; 95% CI 0.6–3.3, respectively). In conclusion, there are no significant differences in clinical outcomes between the two treatment groups during the in-hospital observational period. According to the UPET study, the 6 month mortality rates between patients treated with thrombolysis and heparin are also comparable.

Safety bleedings
It is well known that serious bleeding can occur with the use of fibrinolytic therapy. Levine et al reported an incidence of major haemorrhage of 8.4% and an incidence of fatal haemorrhage of 2.2%, based on 227 patients treated with rt-PA (50–100 mg).[41] When intracranial haemorrhages are considered, incidence rates vary from 1.5%,[44] to 3%.[29,45] When the incidence of bleedings is analysed in the six randomized trials (Table 8.5), significant differences are observed between thrombolysis and heparin. The rate of major bleedings is higher in the thrombolysis (14%) than in heparin (7%) treatment group (RR 1.8; 95% CI 1.04–3.1). In addition, there is a significant 4-fold higher risk of minor bleedings in patients receiving thrombolysis as compared to heparin recipients.

Although all studies included in the pooled analysis are randomized trials concerning patients with confirmed PE, the small numbers of patients in the individual studies and the difference in agents and dose regimens used limits the conclusion of the pooled results and warrants careful interpretations. Nevertheless, the following conclusions can be drawn. Although there are short-term positive findings with surrogate makers in patients treated with fibrinolytic treatments as compared to patients treated with heparin alone, no clear long-term benefits are observed in surrogate markers. When clinical outcome measures such as recurrent venous thromboembolism and mortality are concerned a trend is seen favouring treatment with thrombolysis; however, these results are by far not statistically significant. Together with the significantly increased bleeding risk in patients treated with thrombolysis, fibrinolytic therapy is not considered to be routinely indicated in patients with acute PE.

Table 8.4 The short-term (in-hospital) efficacy of thrombolysis and heparin vs heparin alone for the initial treatment of acute pulmonary embolism as assessed by clinical outcomes.

Study	No. of patients	Treatment regimens		All-cause mortality		PE-related mortality		Recurrent VTE	
		T(+H)	H	T+H	H	T+H	H	T+H	H
UPET (1970)[37]	160	Urokinase 4400 U/kg + 4400 U/kg/h for 12 hours + heparin	Heparin	6/82	7/78	1/82	0/78	6/82	5/78
Levine et al (1990)[41]	58	0.6 mg/kg/2 min rt-PA + heparin	Heparin	1/33	0/25	1/33	0/25	0/33	0/25
PIOPED (1990)[38]	13	40–80 mg/40–90 min rt-PA + heparin	Heparin	1/9	0/4	0/9	0/4	0/9	0/4
PAIMS-2 (1992)[39]	36	100 mg/2 hours, rt-PA + heparin	Heparin	2/20	1/16	0/20	1/16	2/20	1/16
Ly et al (1978)[55]	25	Streptokinase 250 000 IU/20 min +100 000 IU/hour for 72 hours + heparin	Heparin	1/14	2/11	1/14	2/11	na	na
Tibbutt et al (1974)[56]	20	Streptokinase 600 000 IU/30 min + 100 000/hour for 72 hours	Heparin	0/13	1/17	0/13	1/17	na	na
Marini et al (1988)[57]	30	Urokinase 8 000 000 IU/12 hours/day for 3 days 3 300 000 IU/12 hours	Heparin	0/20	0/10	0/20	0/10	0/20	0/10

(continued)

Table 8.4 The short-term (in-hospital) efficacy of thrombolysis and heparin vs heparin alone for the initial treatment of acute pulmonary embolism as assessed by clinical outcomes.—*continued*

Study	No. of patients	Treatment regimens		All-cause mortality		PE-related mortality		Recurrent VTE	
		T(+H)	H	T+H	H	T+H	H	T+H	H
Goldhaber (1993)[40]	101	100 mg/2 hours rt-PA + heparin	Heparin	0/46	2/55	0/46	2/55	0/46	5/55
Total	453	Thrombolysis + heparin	Heparin	11/237 (4.6%)	13/216 (6.0%)	3/237 (1.3%)	6/216 (2.8%)	8/210 (3.8%)	11/188 (5.9%)
Pooled relative risk (95% CI)				1.3 in favour of thrombolysis (0.6–2.5) Test for heterogeneity $p = 0.91$		1.7 in favour of thrombolysis (0.6–5.0) Test for heterogeneity $p = 0.78$		1.4 in favour of thrombolysis (0.6–3.3) Test for heterogeneity $P = 0.25$	

T, thrombolysis; H, heparin; PE, pulmonary embolism; VTE, venous thromboembolism.

Table 8.5 The safety of thrombolysis and heparin vs heparin alone for the initial treatment of acute pulmonary embolism.

Study	No of patients	Treatment regimens		Major bleedings		Intracranial haemorrhages		Minor bleedings	
		T+H	H	T+H	H	T+H	H	T+H	H
UPET (1970)[37]	160	Urokinase + heparin	Heparin	22/82	11/78	0/82	0/78	na	na
Levine et al (1990)[41]	58	0.6 mg/kg/2 min rt-PA + heparin	Heparin	0/33	0/25	0/33	0/25	15/33	1/25
PIOPED (1990)[38]	13	40–80 mg/40–90 min rt-PA + heparin	Heparin	1/9	0/4	0/9	0/4	na	na
PAIMS-2 (1992)[39]	36	100 mg/2 hours rt-PA + heparin	Heparin	3/20	2/16	1/20	0/16	11/20	4/16
Ly et al (1978)[55]	25	Streptokinase 250 000 IU/20 min +100 000 IU/hour for 72 hours + heparin	Heparin	4/14	2/11	na	na	na	na
Goldhaber et al (1993)[40]	101	100 mg/2 hours rt-PA + heparin	Heparin	1/46	0/55	0/46	0/55	3/46	1/55
Total	368	Thrombolysis + heparin	Heparin	31/204 (15.2%)	15/189 (7.9%)	1/190 (0.5%)	0/178 (0%)	29/99 (29.3%)	6/96 (6.3%)
Pooled relative risk (95% CI)				1.8 (1.04–3.1) Test for heterogeneity p = 0.98		2–4 (0.1–55.9)		4.0 (1.8–9.0) Test for heterogeneity p = 0.26	

na, no exact data available; T, thrombolysis; H, heparin.

Massive pulmonary embolism

As described above, there is no role for fibrinolytic therapy in the standard treatment of patients with acute PE. Massive PE with haemodynamic instability is considered to be the only indication for fibrinolytic treatment. Besides non-controlled observations, the only available evidence for this indication is based on a prematurely stopped randomized study by Jerjes-Sanchez et al in which 4 of the 4 patients who received heparin died, whereas 4 of the 4 patients allocated to thrombolysis all survived.[46]

Right ventricular dysfunction

Some reports suggest an expansion of the indication for fibrinolytic therapy in patients with PE to those with 'impending haemodynamic instability' (i.e. patients with adequate blood pressure but who have echocardiographic signs of right ventricular dysfunction).[47,48] About 30–40% of the patients presenting with PE have right ventricular dysfunction. In-hospital as well as long-term (up to 1 year) mortality seems to be increased in these patients. Ribeiro et al and Kasper and colleagues showed that right ventricular dysfunction is associated with a more than 3-fold increase in in-hospital as well as one year total mortality.[49,50] Another recent study showed an increase in PE-related in-hospital mortality between patients with echocardiographic right ventricular dysfunction (5%, 95% CI 0–13%) as compared to those without (0%, 95% CI 0–4%). To reduce the increased mortality rate in PE patients with echocardiographic right ventricular dysfunction, this subset of patients might benefit from more intensive treatment, such as thrombolysis. Thus far, only two non-randomized trials have compared the mortality in haemodynamically stable patients with echocardiographic signs of right ventricular overload receiving thrombolysis and heparin to those receiving heparin alone.[51,52] In the first study, a 30 day mortality rate of 4.7% was observed in the thrombolysis group compared with 11.1% in the heparin group ($p = 0.16$). In contrast, in the other study, 4% of the patients in the thrombolysis group died versus 0% in the heparin group ($p = 0.12$). The percentage of recurrent pulmonary embolism in both groups were similar; however, the frequency of serious bleedings in the thrombolysis group (9.4%) significantly exceeded that in the heparin group (0%). Since these registry data are far from conclusive, the question whether to treat haemodynamically stable patients with echocardiographic signs of right ventricular overload with fibrinolytics remains unresolved and needs to be addressed urgently in a proper randomized study. Recently, such a randomised trial between heparin plus rt-PA and heparin alone in patients with submassive pulmonary embolism has been carried out. With regard to the endpoint treatment escalation, a benefit of thrombolysis was observed. However, no differences between PE-related mortality and recurrent PE were found.[53]

Dose regimen

A task force committee for guidelines on diagnosis and management of acute PE listed all the relevant issues regarding the question which drug or dose regimen is to be preferred.[54] With respect to differences in clinical outcome between the various regimens, no difference in mortality was found between rt-PA, streptokinase or urokinase. However, differences exist in early haemodynamic improvement and bleeding. A 2 hour infusion of 100 mg rt-PA achieves more rapid lysis than urokinase (4400 IU/kg/h) during 12–24 hours; 0.6 mg/kg/15 min rt-PA and 1.5 million IU streptokinase/2 hours. However, the difference between 100 mg rt-PA/2 hours, 0.6 mg/kg/15 min and streptokinase/2 hours is limited to the first hour. Major bleeding complications occurred in 28% of the patients receiving urokinase in 12 hours, in 21–24% of patients receiving 100 mg of rt-PA and in 11% of patients receiving 0.6 mg/kg rt-PA. However, these differences did not reach statistical significance. Thus, no conclusive answer is available to the question which drug must be preferred for the treatment of patients with massive PE. The task force committee suggests that faster haemodynamic improvement may be relevant in the sickest patients, whereas the low incidence of bleeding observed with the 0.6 mg/kg rt-PA bolus injection may be useful in patients with relative contraindications. Goldhaber[47] argues that streptokinase instead of rt-PA might be the preferred drug, since large studies in patients with myocardial infarction showed that the risk of intracranial bleeding appears to be lower in patients treated with 1 500 000 U of streptokinase as compared to patients receiving rt-PA.

Summary: practical guidelines

- There is no indication for fibrinolytic therapy in patients with deep vein thrombosis.
- The indication for fibrinolytic therapy in patients with pulmonary embolism is limited to those patients with massive pulmonary embolism, accompanied with hypotension and/or shock.
- The following drug and dose regimens can be used:
  1. rt-PA 100 mg in 2 hours.
  2. Urokinase 4400 U/kg (loading dose over 10 min), followed by 4400 U/h for 12–24 hours.
  3. Streptokinase 250 000 U (loading dose over 30 min), then 100 000 U/h for 24 hours.
- Fibrinolytic therapy should be instituted after objective testing; that is, high-probability scintigraphy, abnormal spiral computed tomography (CT) or angiography; or in case of a high clinical suspicion combined with evidence of acute cor pulmonale (e.g. shown by echocardiography).

- The use of fibrinolytic therapy in patients with submassive pulmonary embolism (right ventricular dysfunction) is controversial.
- Patients without massive pulmonary embolism should be treated with unfractionated heparin (or low molecular weight heparin). Unfractionated heparin should be started with a loading dose of 5000 U, followed by continuous infusion of 1250 U/hour. Frequent measurements of activated partial thromboplastin time (APTT) are required to prolong the APTT 1.5–2.5 times the normal range. The duration of treatment is at least 5 days and can be stopped when the INR is two times above 2.
- In all patients treatment with vitamin K antagonists is indicated for at least 3 months. Therapeutic treatment aims at an INR between 2 and 3.

References

1. Hull RD, Hirsh J, Carter CJ et al. Pulmonary angiography, ventilation lung scanning, and venography for clinically suspected pulmonary embolism with abnormal perfusion lung scan. Ann Intern Med 1983; **98**:891–9.

2. Kruit WH, de Boer AC, Sing AK, van Roon F. The significance of venography in the management of patients with clinically suspected pulmonary embolism. J Intern Med 1991; **230**:333–9.

3. Huisman MV, Buller HR, Ten Cate JW et al. Unexpected high prevalence of silent pulmonary embolism in patients with deep venous thrombosis. Chest 1989; **95**:498–502.

4. Nordstrom M, Lindblad B, Bergqvist D, Kjellstrom T. A prospective study of the incidence of deep-vein thrombosis within a defined urban population. J Intern Med 1992; **232**:155–60.

5. Prandoni P, Lensing AW, Cogo A et al. The long-term clinical course of acute deep venous thrombosis. Ann Intern Med 1996; **125**:1–7.

6. van den Belt AG, Prins MH, Lensing AW et al. Fixed dose subcutaneous low molecular weight heparins versus adjusted dose unfractionated heparin for venous thromboembolism. Cochrane Database Syst Rev 2000 (2):CD001100.

7. Lindner DJ, Edwards JM, Phinney ES, Taylor LM, Jr, Porter JM. Long-term hemodynamic and clinical sequelae of lower extremity deep vein thrombosis. J Vasc Surg 1986; **4**:436–42.

8. Wells PS, Forster AJ. Thrombolysis in deep vein thrombosis: is there still an indication? Thromb Haemost 2001; **86**:499–508.

9. Robertson BR, Nilsson IM, Nylander G. Thrombolytic effect of streptokinase as evaluated by phlebography of deep venous thrombi of the leg. Acta Chir Scand. 1970; **136**:173–80.

10. Robertson BR, Nilsson IM, Nylander G. Value of streptokinase and heparin in treatment of acute deep venous thrombosis. A coded investigation. Acta Chir Scand 1968; **134**:203–8.

11. Kakkar VV, Flanc C, Howe CT, O'Shea M, Flute PT. Treatment of deep vein thrombosis. A trial of

heparin, streptokinase, and arvin. BMJ 1969; **1**:806–10.

12. Tsapogas MJ, Peabody RA, Wu KT, Karmody AM, Devaraj KT, Eckert C. Controlled study of thrombolytic therapy in deep vein thrombosis. Surgery 1973; **74**:973–84.

13. Elliot MS, Immelman EJ, Jeffery P et al. A comparative randomized trial of heparin versus streptokinase in the treatment of acute proximal venous thrombosis: an interim report of a prospective trial. Br J Surg 1979; **66**:838–43.

14. Arnesen H, Heilo A, Jakobsen E, Ly B, Skaga E. A prospective study of streptokinase and heparin in the treatment of deep vein thrombosis. Acta Med Scand 1978; **203**:457–63.

15. Porter JM, Seaman AJ, Common HH, Rosch J, Eidemiller LR, Calhoun AD. Comparison of heparin and streptokinase in the treatment of venous thrombosis. Am Surg 1975; **41**:511–19.

16. Turpie AG, Levine MN, Hirsh J et al. Tissue plasminogen activator (rt-PA) vs heparin in deep vein thrombosis. Results of a randomized trial. Chest 1990; **97**(suppl 4):172S–5S.

17. Goldhaber SZ, Meyerovitz MF, Green D et al. Randomized controlled trial of tissue plasminogen activator in proximal deep venous thrombosis. Am J Med 1990; **88**:235–40.

18. Verhaeghe R, Besse P, Bounameaux H, Marbet GA. Multicenter pilot study of the efficacy and safety of systemic rt-PA administration in the treatment of deep vein thrombosis of the lower extremities and/or pelvis. Thromb Res 1989; **55**:5–11.

19. Goldhaber SZ, Hirsch DR, MacDougall RC, Polak JF, Creager MA. Bolus recombinant urokinase versus heparin in deep venous thrombosis: a randomized controlled trial. Am Heart J 1996; **132**:314–18.

20. Kiil J, Carvalho A, Sakso P, Nielsen HO. Urokinase or heparin in the management of patients with deep vein thrombosis? Acta Chir Scand 1981; **147**:529–32.

21. Grossman C, McPherson S. Safety and efficacy of catheter-directed thrombolysis for ilio-femoral venous thrombosis. Am J Roentgenol 1999; **172**: 667–72.

22. Mewissen MW, Seabrook GR, Meissner MH, Cynamon J, Labropoulos N, Haughton SH. Catheter-directed thrombolysis for lower extremity deep venous thrombosis: report of a national multicenter registry. Radiology 1999; **211**:39–49.

23. Hansson PO, Welin L, Tibblin G, Eriksson H. Deep vein thrombosis and pulmonary embolism in the general population. 'The Study of Men Born in 1913'. Arch Intern Med 1997; **157**: 1665–70.

24. Goldhaber SZ. Pulmonary embolism. N Engl J Med 1998; **339**:93–104 (Review, see comments).

25. Rubinstein I, Murray D, Hoffstein V. Fatal pulmonary emboli in hospitalized patients. An autopsy study. Arch Intern Med 1988; **148**:1425–6.

26. Barker NW, Nygaard KK, Walters W, Priestly JT. A statistical study of postoperative venous thrombosis and pulmonary embolism: 1. Incidence in various types of operations. Proceedings of the Staff Meetings of the Mayo Clinic 1940; **15**:769–73.

27. Short DS. A survey of pulmonary embolism in a general hospital. BMJ 1952; **i**:790–6.

28. Barrit DW, Jordan SC. Anticoagulant drugs in the treatment of pulmonary embolism. A

controlled trial. Lancet 1960; **1**:1309–12.

29. Goldhaber SZ, Visani L, De Rosa M. Acute pulmonary embolism: clinical outcomes in the International Cooperative Pulmonary Embolism Registry (ICOPER). Lancet 1999; **353**: 1386–9.

30. Van Beek EJ, Kuijer PM, Buller HR et al. The clinical course of patients with suspected pulmonary embolism. Arch Intern Med 1997; **157**:2593–8.

31. Carson JL, Kelley MA, Duff A et al. The clinical course of pulmonary embolism. N Engl J Med 1992; **326**:1240–5.

32. Brandjes DP, Heijboer H, Buller HR, de Rijk M, Jagt H, Ten Cate JW. Acenocoumarol and heparin compared with acenocoumarol alone in the initial treatment of proximal-vein thrombosis. N Engl J Med 1992; **327**:1485–9.

33. Hull RD, Raskob GE, Rosenbloom D et al. Heparin for 5 days as compared with 10 days in the initial treatment of proximal venous thrombosis. N Engl J Med 1990; **322**:1260–4 (See comments).

34. Hirsh J. Oral anticoagulant drugs. N Engl J Med 1991; **324**:1865–75 (Review, see comments).

35. van der Heijden JF, Prins MH, Buller HR. Low-molecular-weight heparins: are they interchangeable? Haemostasis 2000; **30**(suppl 2):148–57.

36. Goldhaber SZ, Vaughan DE, Markis JE et al. Acute pulmonary embolism treated with tissue plasminogen activator. Lancet [JID–2985213R] 1986; **2**:886–9.

37. Urokinase Pulmonary Embolism Trial (UPET). Phase 1 results: a cooperative study. JAMA 1970; **214**:2163–72.

38. PIOPED investigators.Tissue plasminogen activator for the treatment of acute pulmonary embolism. A collaborative study by the PIOPED Investigators. Chest 1990; **97**:528–33.

39. Dalla-Volta S, Palla A, Santolicandro A et al. PAIMS 2: alteplase combined with heparin versus heparin in the treatment of acute pulmonary embolism. Plasminogen activator Italian multicenter study 2. J Am Coll Cardiol 1992; **20**:520–6.

40. Goldhaber SZ, Haire WD, Feldstein ML et al. Alteplase versus heparin in acute pulmonary embolism: randomised trial assessing right-ventricular function and pulmonary perfusion. Lancet 1993; **341**:507–11.

41. Levine M, Hirsh J, Weitz J et al. A randomized trial of a single bolus dosage regimen of recombinant tissue plasminogen activator in patients with acute pulmonary embolism. Chest 1990; **98**:1473–9.

42. Come PC, Kim D, Parker JA, Goldhaber SZ, Braunwald E, Markis JE. Early reversal of right ventricular dysfunction in patients with acute pulmonary embolism after treatment with intravenous tissue plasminogen activator. J Am Coll Cardiol 1987; **10**:971–8.

43. Konstantinides S, Tiede N, Geibel A, Olschewski M, Kasper W. Comparison of alteplase versus heparin for resolution of major pulmonary embolism. Am J Cardiol 1998; **82**:966–70.

44. Meyer G, Gisselbrecht M, Diehl JL, Journois D, Sors H. Incidence and predictors of major hemorrhagic complications from thrombolytic therapy in patients with massive pulmonary embolism. Am J Med 1998; **105**:472–7.

45. Dalen JE, Alpert JS, Hirsh J. Thrombolytic therapy for pulmonary embolism: is it effective? Is it safe? When is it indicated? Arch Intern Med 1997; **157**:2550–6 (Review, see comments).

46. Jerjes-Sanchez C, Ramirez-Rivera A, de Lourdes GM et al. Streptokinase and heparin versus heparin alone in massive pulmonary embolism: a randomized controlled trial. J Thromb Thrombolysis 1995; **2**:227–9.

47. Goldhaber SZ. Thrombolysis in pulmonary embolism: a large-scale clinical trial is overdue. Circulation [JID–0147763] 2001; **104**:2876–8.

48. Goldhaber SZ. Thrombolysis in pulmonary embolism: a debatable indication. Thromb Haemost [JID–7608063] 2001; **86**:444–51.

49. Ribeiro A, Lindmarker P, Juhlin-Dannfelt A, Johnsson H, Jorfeldt L. Echocardiography Doppler in pulmonary embolism: right ventricular dysfunction as a predictor of mortality rate. Am Heart J 1997; **134**:479–87.

50. Kasper W, Konstantinides S, Geibel A, Tiede N, Krause T, Just H. Prognostic significance of right ventricular afterload stress detected by echocardiography in patients with clinically suspected pulmonary embolism. Heart 1997; **77**:346–9.

51. Konstantinides S, Geibel A, Olschewski M et al. Association between thrombolytic treatment and the prognosis of hemodynamically stable patients with major pulmonary embolism: results of a multicenter registry. Circulation 1997; **96**:882–8 (See comments).

52. Hamel E, Pacouret G, Vincentelli D et al. Thrombolysis or heparin therapy in massive pulmonary embolism with right ventricular dilation: results from a 128-patient monocenter registry. Chest [JID–0231335] 2001; **120**:120–5.

53. Konstantinides S, Geibel A, Heusel G, Heinrich F, Kasper W, the Management Strategies and Prognosis of Pulmonary Embolism–3 Trial Investigators. Heparin plus alteplase compared with heparin alone in patients with submassive pulmonary embolism. N Engl J Med 2002; **347**:1143–1150.

54. Guidelines on diagnosis and management of acute pulmonary embolism. Task Force on Pulmonary Embolism, European Society of Cardiology. Eur Heart J [JID–8006263] 2000; **21**:1301–36.

55. Ly B, Arnesen H, Eie H, Hol R. A controlled clinical trial of streptokinase and heparin in the treatment of major pulmonary embolism. Acta Med Scand 1978; **203**:465–70.

56. Tibbutt DA, Davies JA, Anderson JA et al. Comparison by controlled clinical trial of streptokinase and heparin in treatment of life-threatening pulmonary embolism. BMJ 1974; **1**:343–7.

57. Marini C, Di Ricco G, Rossi G, Rindi M, Palla R, Giuntini C. Fibrinolytic effects of urokinase and heparin in acute pulmonary embolism: a randomized clinical trial. Respiration 1988; **54**:162–73.

9

General principles of fibrinolytic therapy in ischaemic stroke

Peter D Schellinger and Werner Hacke

Introduction

Stroke is the third most common cause of death in the industrialized nations, after myocardial infarction and cancer, and the single most common reason for permanent disability.[1] Up to 85% of all strokes are of ischaemic origin and mostly due to blockage of a cerebral artery by a blood clot.[2] After introduction of thrombolytic therapy for the treatment of acute myocardial infarction in the early 1990s, major trials for the evaluation of this new therapeutic approach to ischaemic stroke were initiated.[3] Occlusion of a brain vessel leads to a critical reduction in cerebral perfusion and, within minutes, to ischaemic infarction with a central infarct core of irreversibly damaged brain tissue with an area of surrounding critical hypoperfusion of varying size (the ischaemic penumbra), which can be salvaged by rapid restoration of blood flow.[4,5] Therefore, the underlying rationale for the introduction and application of thrombolytic agents is the lysis of an obliterating thrombus and subsequent re-establishment of cerebral blood flow by cerebrovascular recanalization.[6]

Initial patient assessment

In addition to standard care in acutely ill patients, such as stabilization of vital parameters, an accurate assessment of the patient's neurological status is essential.[5] With the use of standard stroke scales, such as the US National Institutes of Health Stroke Scale (NIHSS) or the Scandinavian Stroke Scale,[7,8] stroke severity can be rapidly graded, with the goal of excluding small as well as large infarctions from a potentially hazardous therapy. Information about the time-point of stroke onset is crucial as the therapeutic time window is small. Besides the usual contraindications for thrombolytic therapy, in general, intracranial haemorrhage (ICH) and severe microangiopathy must be excluded by imaging procedures, such as computed tomography (CT) or magnetic resonance imaging (MRI).[7,9]

Evidence of an occluded vessel by Doppler ultrasound, CT, MRI or digital subtraction angiography should be established, at least when thrombolysis is performed later than 3 hours after symptom onset. However, the evidence is not yet required for the indication of thrombolytic therapy and was not an inclusion criterion in any of the intravenous thrombolysis trials. Overall, the saying 'time is brain' holds true; therefore, a rapid work-up of the patient who is a potential candidate for thrombolytic therapy is mandatory.

Intravenous thrombolysis for acute ischaemic stroke

In 1933, Tillet and Garner reported that streptococci released a substance that dissolved blood clots.[10] The first anecdotal report of thrombolytic therapy for ischaemic stroke dates back to the early 1960s.[11] Three trials in the early 1980s investigated the effect of low-dose intravenous urokinase for the therapy of acute (5 or 14 days after stroke onset) ischaemic stroke.[12-14] In the early 1990s, three small trials of intravenous thrombolysis with rt-PA (alteplase) were carried out.[15-17] These trials, although not large enough to prove efficacy, certainly demonstrated the feasibility of early thrombolytic therapy and also suggested a reasonable degree of safety and a potential benefit.

The streptokinase trials

One pilot study and three large, randomized, controlled trials investigated the efficacy of streptokinase for acute ischaemic stroke.[18-21] In summary, all of the trials using streptokinase for acute ischaemic stroke were prematurely stopped due to a high rate of early death, mostly due to intracerebral haemorrhage (ICH), and also because of lack of benefit at outcome in a meta-analysis.[22] In all the streptokinase trials there were 92 (95% CI 65–120) additional fatal ICH per 1000 treated patients (OR 6.03; 95% CI 3.47–10.47).[23] The higher bleeding rate may be due to the pharmacological properties of streptokinase rather than, for example, rt-PA, additional anticoagulation (MAST-E), a small number of patients treated within 3 hours, and a high dose of 1.5 MU streptokinase, which is identical to the dose used in myocardial infarction (MI). The rt-PA studies (see below), however, chose approximately two-thirds the dose used in MI. Other side effects of streptokinase are a decrease in systolic blood pressure of more than 20 mmHg in 33% (only 6% in the placebo group) as well as anaphylaxis in 2.2% of the patients. Therefore, intravenous administration of streptokinase, outside the setting of a clinical investigation, is dangerous and contraindicated for the management of patients with ischaemic stroke.

The rt-PA trials

In 1995, the results of the ECASS I and NINDS trials of intravenous rt-PA for acute ischaemic stroke were published,[7,9,24] followed by ECASS II in 1998,[24] and ATLANTIS in 1999.[25] These four trials randomized a total of 2657 patients to treatment with placebo (N = 1316 patients) or intravenous rt-PA (N = 1341 patients) within 0–3 hours (NINDS), 3–5 hours (ATLANTIS) or 0–6 hours (ECASS I and II) after symptom onset. All four studies required a baseline computed tomographic (CT) scan to exclude ICH and, except for the NINDS study, all the others also established CT exclusion criteria, such as major early signs of infarction. All trials used the 0.9 mg/kg bodyweight dose up to a maximum of 90 mg rt-PA, except ECASS I, in which 1.1 mg/kg up to a maximum dose of 100 mg was given. Ten per cent of the total dose was given as a bolus; the remainder was infused over 1 hour in all four trials.

NINDS

The NINDS trial (National Institute of Neurological Disorders and Stroke) randomized 624 patients (312 placebo, 312 intravenous rt-PA) within a time window of 3 hours after stroke symptom onset.[7] A good outcome was defined as an NIHSS score of ≤ 1 Glasgow Outcome Score (GOS) = 1, Barthel Index (BI) ≥ 95 and Modified Rankin Scale (MRS) ≤ 1. The median baseline NIHSS score was 14 (rt-PA group) versus 15 (placebo group). The long-term clinical benefit of rt-PA was confirmed in all single scores as well as in the global test: BI [50% vs 38%, OR 1.6 (1.1–2.5), p = 0.026]; MRS [39% vs 26%, OR 1.7 (1.1–2.5), p = 0.019]; GOS [44% vs 32%, OR 1.6 (1.1–2.5), p = 0.025]; NIHSS [31% vs 20%, OR 1.7 (1.0–2.8), p = 0.033]; and combined end-point [OR 1.7 (1.2–2.6), p = 0.008]. For every 100 patients treated with rt-PA, an additional 11–13 will have a favourable outcome as compared to 100 not treated with rt-PA. Symptomatic ICH occurred in 6.4% of rt-PA patients compared to only 0.6% of placebo patients (p < 0.001). After publication of the NINDS trial in 1996, rt-PA received US Food and Drug Administration (FDA) approval for the treatment of acute ischaemic stroke in the 3 hour time window.

ECASS I

ECASS I recruited 620 patients for treatment either with 1.1 mg/kg rt-PA or placebo within 6 hours after stroke onset.[9] Patients with a severe neurological deficit, only mild or improving stroke symptoms, or CT signs of early infarction exceeding 33% of the middle cerebral artery (MCA) territory were excluded. Primary end-points included a difference of 15 points in the BI and 1 point in the MRS at 90 days in favour of rt-PA. The median

NIHSS score at baseline was 13 (rt-PA patients) and 12 (placebo group), respectively. ECASS I was the first trial of thrombolysis to use CT exclusion criteria.[26–29] Despite these predefined parameters there were 109 protocol violations in ECASS I (17.4%), 66 (11%) of which were CT protocol violations and 52 (8.4%) of these due to maldetection of early infarct signs. There was no difference in the primary endpoints in the intention to treat (ITT) analysis, while the target population (TP) analysis (protocol violaters excluded) revealed a significant difference in the MRS in favour of rt-PA-treated patients (p = 0.035). There was a significant increase in parenchymal ICH (19.8% vs 6.5%, p < 0.001) and a significant inverse relationship between protocol violation in rt-PA patients and 7 day survival. A *post hoc* analysis of the ECASS I 3 hour cohort (N = 87 patients) did not reveal a significant difference between rt-PA and placebo group outcomes.[30]

ECASS II

A total of 800 patients (409 rt-PA, 391 placebo) were randomized to treatment with either 0.9 mg/kg rt-PA or placebo within 6 hours after stroke symptom onset.[24] The primary end-point was the MRS at 90 days, dichotomized for favourable (score 0–1) and unfavourable (score 2–6) outcome and for an alternative dichotomization into independent versus death and dependent outcome (MRS 0–2 vs 3–6). Baseline median NIHSS was 11 in both groups. There was no difference in mortality (10.5% vs 10.7%) with a larger number of fatal ICH in the rt-PA group (11 vs 2 patients) as opposed to a larger number of deaths due to space-occupying brain oedema (8 vs 17 patients). The primary end-point was negative for rt-PA (MRS 0–1: 40.3% vs 36.6%; Δ = 3.7%; p = 0.277), while the alternative dichotomization showed a significant advantage for patients treated with rt-PA (MRS 0–2: 54.3% vs 46.0%; Δ = 8.3%; p = 0.024). Symptomatic ICH occurred in 36 (8.8%) rt-PA patients and 13 (3.4%) placebo-treated patients. Interestingly, there was a high number of benign spontaneous disease courses in the placebo group (36.6%), which is larger than the favourable outcome rate in the ECASS I rt-PA group (35.9%). Furthermore, a comparison of the 3 hour cohorts of ECASS I and II and NINDS demonstrates a surprisingly high number of favourable outcomes among the placebo group patients in ECASS II (ECASS I rt-PA: 38.5%; NINDS rt-PA: 38.7%; ECASS II placebo: 37.7%). Whether this is due to general improvements in the treatment of acute stroke patients, the less severe baseline deficit, or other factors is unclear. ECASS II was a clinically highly relevant study and showed that treatment of ischaemic stroke with rt-PA in a time window of less than 6 hours may lead to an improved outcome if given to selected patients in experienced centres.

ATLANTIS

The ATLANTIS study began in 1991 and originally was designed to assess efficacy and safety of thrombolytic therapy with rt-PA within 0–6 hours after stroke symptom onset.[25] In 1993, the time window was changed due to safety concerns to 0–5 hours and restarted as ATLANTIS part B (ITT), only to be further modified in 1996 to a 3–5 hour window (TP) after rt-PA had been approved by the FDA. There were no differences on any of the primary (34% vs 32%, p = 0.65) or secondary functional outcome measures. Treatment with rt-PA significantly increased the rate of symptomatic ICH (7.0% vs 1.1%, p < 0.001). As in ECASS II (median baseline NIHSS: 11 points), the median baseline NIHSS score was substantially lower than in the NINDS trial (10 vs 14 points), which (as in ECASS II) may have led to a better than expected outcome in the placebo group.

Meta-analyses

A search of the literature revealed two large meta-analyses.[23,31,32] The first meta-analysis by Hacke et al (1999) covered the NINDS study and both ECASS trials, with a total of 2044 patients (1034 rt-PA patients vs 1010 placebo patients).[31] The authors assessed the benefit of rt-PA and dichotomized the outcome into dependent versus independent or dead (MRS 0–2 vs 3–6) and favourable versus unfavourable (MRS 0–1 vs MRS 2–6). ICH occurred significantly more often in patients receiving rt-PA (144/1034 vs 43/1010; OR 3.23; CI 2.39–4.37), and was slightly less increased in the 3 hour time window and at the lower dosage (41/393 vs 15/389; OR 2.68; CI 1.56–4.62). There was no significant difference in mortality between rt-PA and placebo (OR 1.07; CI 0.84–1.36) but a slight trend towards a lower mortality in the 0.9 mg/kg and 3 hour group (OR 0.91; CI 0.63–1.32). rt-pA led to a 37% reduction in death and dependence, regardless of dose and time window (OR 0.63; CI 0.53–0.76). If treated with the lower dose and within 3 hours the chance of an unfavourable outcome was reduced by 45% (OR 0.55; CI 0.41–0.72). For every 1000 patients treated with either dose there are 90 fewer patients who are dead or disabled but 96 haemorrhages more than expected with placebo. Conversely, for 1000 patients treated with 0.9 mg/kg and within 3 hours, there are 65 additional ICH and 140 fewer patients dead or disabled. The number needed to treat (NNT) for all doses and time windows is 11; for the 3 hour and 0.9 mg/kg group it is 7. These numbers are far better than the NNT for thrombolysis in myocardial infarctions, which are 30–40 (Fig. 9.1).[31]

Wardlaw et al (2000) included in their Cochrane Library meta-analysis all randomized trials of thrombolysis, regardless of time window, dosage, administration route and substance.[23,32] Symptomatic and fatal ICH were significantly more common as a result of thrombolytic therapy

Study	rt-PA n / N	Placebo n / N	OR (95% CI Fixed)	OR (95% CI Fixed)
Mortality				
ECASS I	69 / 313	48 / 307		1.52 (1.02–2.27)
ECASS II	43 / 409	42 / 391		0.98 (0.62–1.53)
NINDS	54 / 312	64 / 312		0.81 (0.54–1.21)
Subtotal (95% CI)	166 / 1034	154 / 1010		1.07 (0.84–1.36)
Chi-square 4.91 (df = 2) Z = 0.55				
All intracranial haemorrhage				
ECASS I	62 / 313	20 / 307		3.18 (2.00–5.06)
ECASS II	48 / 409	12 / 391		3.48 (2.06–5.89)
NINDS	34 / 312	11 / 312		3.00 (1.64–5.51)
Subtotal (95% CI)	144 / 1034	43 / 1010		3.23 (2.39–4.37)
Chi-square 0.14 (df = 2) Z = 7.61				

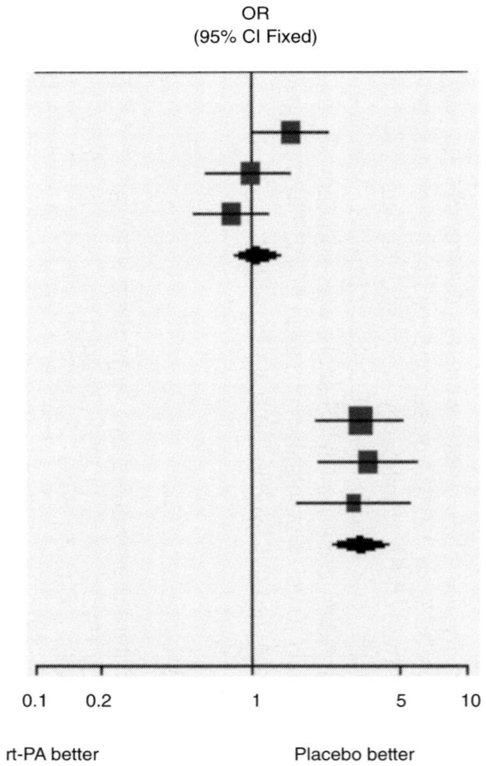

0.1   0.2   1   5   10

rt-PA better   Placebo better

Figure 9.1a
Meta-analysis: death or intracranial haemorrhage (ICH) < 6 hour time window.

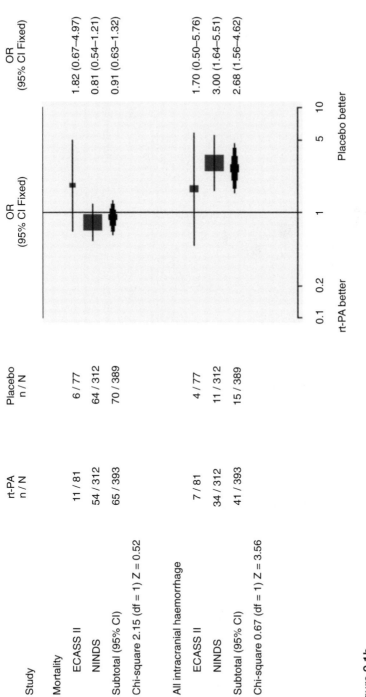

Study	rt-PA n/N	Placebo n/N	OR (95% CI Fixed)
Mortality			
ECASS II	11 / 81	6 / 77	1.82 (0.67–4.97)
NINDS	54 / 312	64 / 312	0.81 (0.54–1.21)
Subtotal (95% CI)	65 / 393	70 / 389	0.91 (0.63–1.32)
Chi-square 2.15 (df = 1) Z = 0.52			
All intracranial haemorrhage			
ECASS II	7 / 81	4 / 77	1.70 (0.50–5.76)
NINDS	34 / 312	11 / 312	3.00 (1.64–5.51)
Subtotal (95% CI)	41 / 393	15 / 389	2.68 (1.56–4.62)
Chi-square 0.67 (df = 1) Z = 3.56			

0.1   0.2   1   5   10

rt-PA better   Placebo better

Figure 9.1b

Meta-analysis: death or intracranial haemorrhage (ICH) < 3 hour time window.

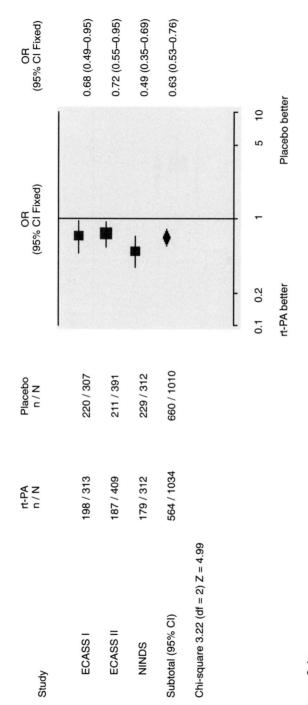

Figure 9.1c

Meta-analysis: Modified Rankin Scale (MRS) 0–2 versus 3–6 < 6 hour time window.

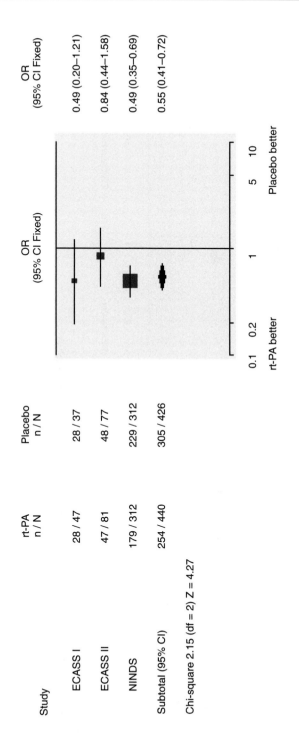

Study	rt-PA n / N	Placebo n / N	OR (95% CI Fixed)	OR (95% CI Fixed)
ECASS I	28 / 47	28 / 37		0.49 (0.20–1.21)
ECASS II	47 / 81	48 / 77		0.84 (0.44–1.58)
NINDS	179 / 312	229 / 312		0.49 (0.35–0.69)
Subtotal (95% CI)	254 / 440	305 / 426		0.55 (0.41–0.72)

Chi-square 2.15 (df = 2) Z = 4.27

Figure 9.1d

Meta-analysis: Modified Rankin Scale (MRS) 0–2 versus 3–6 < 3 hour time window.

Study	rt-PA n / N	Placebo n / N	OR (95% CI Fixed)	OR (95% CI Fixed)
ECASS I	198 / 313	220 / 307		0.68 (0.49–0.95)
ECASS II	244 / 409	248 / 391		0.85 (0.64–1.13)
NINDS	179 / 312	229 / 312		0.49 (0.35–0.69)
Subtotal (95% CI)	621 / 1034	697 / 1010		0.68 (0.56–0.81)

Chi-square 6.08 (df = 2) Z = 4.21

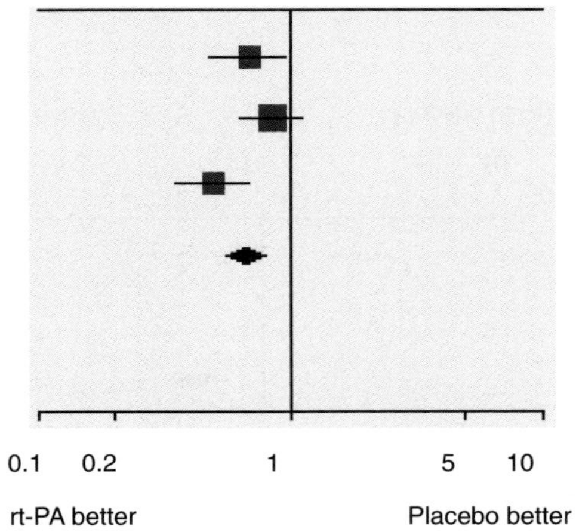

0.1   0.2   1   5   10

rt-PA better   Placebo better

Figure 9.1e

Meta-analysis: Modified Rankin Scale (MRS) 0–1 versus 2–6 < 6 hour time window.

(symptomatic ICH: OR 3.53; CI 2.79–4.45, p < 0.000001; fatal ICH: OR 4.15; CI 2.96–5.84). This translates into 70 additional instances of symptomatic ICH for patients receiving thrombolysis and 29/1000 (OR 3.2) additional instances of fatal ICH in rt-PA patients but 92/1000 (OR 6.03) additional ICH in those patients receiving streptokinase as opposed to placebo. Despite this, thrombolytic therapy, administered up to 6 hours after ischaemic stroke, significantly reduced death or dependence at the end of follow-up (55.2% vs 59.7%, OR 0.83; CI 0.73–0.94, p = 0.0015), which is equivalent to 44 fewer patients being dead or dependent per 1000 treated (CI 15–73). For patients treated with rt-PA only, the OR was 0.79 (CI 0.68–0.92, p = 0.001) or 57 deaths/dependence prevented per 1000 patients treated (CI 20–93). When treatment was given within 3 hours after stroke onset, there was an even better risk reduction for dependency or death (55.2% vs 68.3%; OR 0.58; CI 0.46–0.74, p = 0.00001) or 126 fewer dead or dependent patients per 1000 treated. The difference of benefit of rt-PA in the 0–3 hour window or 3–6 hour window was nonsignificant but showed a trend towards better improvement with early therapy (OR 0.7 vs 0.76). The authors conclude that the significant increase in early death and fatal and non-fatal symptomatic ICH are offset by the significant reduction of disability in survivors. Therapy with rt-PA is associated with less risk and more benefit than with other substances.

Phase IV trials of intravenous thrombolysis and cost aspects

Following FDA approval of rt-PA for intravenous thrombolytic therapy in June 1996, the rate of thrombolysis remained fairly constant until the end of 1998.[31] At most centres where thrombolysis is performed, the NINDS protocol is used; many of these centres also use the ECASS-CT criteria of early infarction. Overall, it is estimated that only 1% of all ischaemic stroke patients and only 2% of the time-eligible (3 hour window) are treated with rt-PA. Also, the reported outcome and complication rates seem to be similar to the NINDS trial in most instances. In Cologne, approximately 22% of the patients that arrive within 3 hours after symptom onset (5% of all ischaemic stroke patients) receive thrombolysis.[33] This rate was achieved after a joint effort was initiated between emergency caregivers, internists and neurologists, and the referral system optimized. The average door-to-needle time in Cologne is 48 min. A total of 150 patients treated within 3 hours were re-evaluated after 12 months.[34] Then, 41% of the patients had an MRS score of ≤ 1 and 52% of ≤ 2. In Houston, 30 patients were treated prospectively after the NINDS protocol.[35] Of all patients hospitalized with ischaemic stroke, 6%

received rt-PA at the university hospital and 1.1% at the community hospitals, the average door-to-needle time was 1 hour 40 min. The STARS (Standard Treatment with Alteplase to Reverse Stroke) study was a prospective, multicentre study of consecutive patients, who received rt-PA according to NINDS criteria.[36] Here, 389 patients received rt-PA within 2 hours 44 min, and the median baseline NIHSS score was 13. The 30 day mortality rate was 13%, 35% of patients had very favourable outcomes (MRS ≤ 1), and 43% were functionally independent (MRS ≤ 2) at day 30. Another 3.3% of the patients experienced symptomatic intracerebral haemorrhage (ICH), which was fatal in 7 patients. Asymptomatic ICH was seen in 8.2%. The mean door-to-needle time was 1 hour 36 min. The authors conclude that favourable clinical outcomes and low rates of symptomatic ICH can be achieved using rt-PA for stroke treatment, while the time effort for emergency evaluation may leave room for logistic improvement. Another study yielded different results.[37] A total of 29 hospitals in the metropolitan area of Cleveland, Ohio, prospectively assessed the rate of rt-PA use, rate of ICH and outcomes in 3948 stroke patients: 70 patients (1.8%) admitted with ischaemic stroke received rt-PA, 16 patients (22%) experienced ICH; 11 of these patients (15.7%) had a symptomatic ICH (of which 6 were fatal), and 50% had deviations from national treatment guidelines. In-hospital mortality was significantly higher (p < 0.001) among patients treated with rt-PA (15.7%) than in patients not receiving rt-PA (5.1%). The fact that blood pressure guidelines were followed in only 47.8% and that the base-line NIHSS was only documented in 40% of the patients illustrates that intravenous thrombolysis, though an effective therapy, should be performed at experienced centres only and may explain the substantially higher rate of mortality and ICH in this study compared to other investigators.

The costs associated with intravenous thrombolytic therapy will be a factor in determining the extent of its utilization. In NINDS, the average length of stay was significantly shorter in rt-PA-treated patients than in placebo-treated patients (10.9 vs 12.4 days; p = 0.02) and more rt-PA patients were discharged to home than to in-patient rehabilitation or a nursing home (48% vs 36%; p = 0.002). An increase in hospitalization costs of $1.7 million is matched by a decrease in rehabilitation costs of $1.4 million and nursing home costs of $4.8 million per 1000 treated patients with a greater than 90% probability of cost savings. The estimated impact on long-term health outcomes was 564 quality-adjusted life-years saved over 30 years per 1000 patients, which makes a net cost savings to the health care system likely. With growing experience and better training of emergency medicine personnel, internists and neurologists throughout all stroke services, the efficacy of intravenous thrombolytic therapy may even improve and the time window may be routinely extended to 6 hours.

Intra-arterial thrombolysis for acute ischaemic stroke

The delivery of thrombolytic agents locally has the advantage of providing a higher concentration of the particular thrombolytic agent where it is needed while minimizing the concentration systemically. Hence, local intra-arterial thrombolysis has the potential for greater efficacy with regard to arterial recanalization rates and greater safety with regard to lower risk of haemorrhage. Grade of vessel occlusion is usually assessed with the Thrombolysis in Myocardial Infarction (TIMI) flow grade, where TIMI-0 is complete occlusion, TIMI-1 minimal perfusion, TIMI-2 partial flow (recanalization) and TIMI-3 complete flow (recanalization).[38] The technique involves performing a cerebral arteriogram, localizing the occluding clot, navigating a microcatheter to the site of the clot and administering the lytic agent (urokinase, rt-PA or pro-urokinase) at or inside the clot with or without mechanical dissolution of the thrombus. Results of several case series on local thrombolysis in the carotid artery territory have been promising, although not convincing.[39–53] The combined partial or complete recanalization rate for these patients was 75%, clearly higher than that demonstrated in the angiography-based intravenous studies (approximately 55%). The most feared complication of local intra-arterial therapy for stroke, as for intravenous thrombolytic therapy, is intracerebral haemorrhage (ICH). Other complications of intra-arterial thrombolysis include arterial intracranial embolization, subarachnoid haemorrhage, arterial perforation, secondary embolization, haemorrhagic infarction, groin haematoma, and retroperitoneal haematoma. These complications occur infrequently, certainly in less than 5% for all the series *in toto*. One drawback of intra-arterial in contrast to intravenous thrombolysis is the considerable time delay to angiography, and from initiation of angiography to clot lysis.[39,40,53] There are few data at present to support the combined use of intravenous and intra-arterial thrombolysis with rt-PA.[54] The underlying rationale for this approach is the reduction of any delay for thrombolysis, while still having the higher recanalization rate and proven larger time window for therapy with the intra-arterial approach. However, this protocol should be limited to clinical investigations.

PROACT I

PROACT I was a randomized phase II trial of recombinant pro-urokinase (rpro-UK) versus placebo in patients with angiographically documented proximal middle cerebral artery occlusion.[55] Angiography was performed after exclusion of ICH by CT. Patients displaying TIMI grade 0 or 1 occlusion of the M1 or M2 middle cerebral artery received either rpro-UK (6 mg) or placebo over 120 min into the proximal thrombus face. Recanalization efficacy was assessed at the end of the 2 hour infusion and symptomatic

ICH at 24 hours. A total of 26 patients received rpro-UK and 14 placebo at a median of 5.5 hours from symptom onset. Recanalization was significantly associated with rpro-UK ($p = 0.0085$) and TIMI-3 recanalization was achieved in 5 rpro-UK patients, as opposed to none of the placebo patients. ICH occurred in 15.4% of the rpro-UK-treated patients and 7.1% of the placebo-treated patients (non-significant).

PROACT II

PROACT II, a randomized, controlled, multicentre, open-label clinical trial with blinded follow-up, aimed to determine the clinical efficacy and safety of 9 mg intra-arterial rpro-UK/2 hours in patients with acute stroke of less than 6 hours duration caused by middle cerebral artery (MCA) occlusion.[56] Mechanical disruption of the clot was not permitted. After 1 hour a control angiogram was performed and the catheter readjusted to the proximal thrombus face. The primary outcome was the rate of patients with an MRS of ≤ 2 at 90 days. A total of 121 rpro-UK and 59 control patients with a median baseline NIHSS of 17 points were included for ITT analysis: 40% of rpro-UK patients and 25% of control patients had an MRS of 2 or less at day 90 (absolute benefit 15%, relative benefit 58%, NNT = 7; $p = 0.04$). Mortality was 25% for the rpro-UK group and 27% for the control group ($p = 0.8$.) The recanalization rate was 66% for the rpro-UK group and 18% for the control group ($p < 0.001$); TIMI-3 recanalization rates were 19% and 2%, respectively ($p < 0.003$).

Thus, intra-arterial thrombolytic therapy of acute MCA occlusion with 9 mg/2 hours significantly improves outcome if administered within 6 hours after stroke onset. Seven patients need to be treated in order to prevent one patient from death or dependence. The higher rate of symptomatic ICH (10.2% in PROACT II vs 8.8% in ECASS II, 6.4% in NINDS and 7.2% in ATLANTIS) is very well explained by the far larger baseline severity of stroke in PROACT II. According to the Cochrane meta-analysis, combining PROACT I and II data there is a 0.55 OR (CI 0.31–1.00) for death or disability, an OR of 2.39 (CI 0.88–6.47) for early symptomatic ICH (7–10 days) and an OR of 0.75 (CI 0.4–1.42) for death from all causes at follow-up.[34] Although recanalization rates may be superior with intra-arterial (66%) than with intravenous (≈55%) thrombolysis and may even be increased by careful mechanical disruption of a thrombus, in addition to the lytic effect of the drug, a limited availability of centres with 24 hours a day, 7 days a week interventional neuroradiology service may restrict the use of this therapy. On the other hand, the clinically more severe strokes may benefit even more from an intra-arterial than an intravenous approach. Furthermore, the time to eventual recanalization may be substantially shorter with intra-arterial thrombolysis. The results of PROACT II did not suffice for FDA approval. Another (partly stroke MRI based) study of intra-arterial pro-urokinase for acute stroke within 6 hours (PROACT III) is underway.

In brief, vertebrobasilar distribution cerebral infarction has been of particular interest to centres experienced with local intra-arterial thrombolysis. Mortality of vertebrobasilar thromboembolism is high, with overall rates of approximately 70–80%. Successful recanalization, however, was associated with a survival rate of 55–75%, as opposed to 0–10% in persistent or untreated basilar artery occlusion.[57,58] Two-thirds of the survivors after recanalization had a favourable outcome; all survivors in the untreated group were moderately disabled. The natural disease course of vertebrobasilar occlusion has a grim prognosis. Intra-arterial thrombolysis and/or percutaneous transluminal angioplasty (PTA) with or without stenting to date is the only life-saving therapy that has demonstrated benefit with regard to mortality and outcome, albeit not in a randomized trial. However, sufficient data are available to justify intra-arterial thrombolytic therapy in the light of mortality and disability in these patients. The time window for thrombolysis in the posterior circulation has not been established but may be up to and even exceed 12 hours. Presence or absence of vertebrobasilar vessel occlusion can be safely, noninvasively and rapidly established by CT (or MRI) angiography before a neuroradiological intervention is initiated.[59]

Diagnostic imaging and thrombolytic therapy

It has been generally accepted that computed tomography (CT) can demonstrate early infarct signs within the first 2 to 6 hours after stroke. The most common early infarct sign is a frequently subtle grey matter and/or cortical hypodensity.[27–29,60] Other early infarct signs include the loss of the insular ribbon,[61] sulcal effacement due to early oedema in 12–41% of stroke patients,[27–29,62] and the hyperdense middle cerebral artery sign (HMCAS) in 40–60% of patients with angiographically proven middle cerebral artery (MCA) occlusion.[26,63–65] There is an association between the size of early hypodensities and the risk of a secondary haemorrhage,[66] and clinical outcome.[26] ECASS I and II showed that in patients with a small area of hypoattenuation (< 33% of the MCA territory), treatment increased the chance of a good clinical outcome, while rt-PA in patients with a large area of hypoattenuation (> 33% of the MCA territory) had no benefit but increased the risk for a fatal brain haemorrhage.[28] While several studies have shown the usefulness of early CT findings (especially after training) in selecting patients before intravenous thrombolytic therapy,[29] other studies demonstrated that physicians, including general radiologists and neurologists, do not uniformly achieve a sufficient level of sensitivity for identifying CT contraindications for thrombolytic therapy.[67] Computed tomographic angiography (CTA) can provide additional information on stenoses or occlusions in the basal arteries of the brain,[68] as non-ionic contrast material does not affect infarction volume or worsen the symptoms of cerebral ischaemia.[69] In addition to the assessment of a major vessel occlusion, CTA has the potential to deliver information about the quality of the collateral circulation as contrast enhancement in arterial branches beyond the occlusion occurs in those patients.[68,70]

The need is evident for a comprehensive diagnostic tool with which all the important pathophysiological aspects of hyperacute stroke can be investigated. Such a method must answer five decisive questions:

1. Where and how large is the actual area of irreversible ischaemic brain damage?
2. How old is the infarction?
3. Is there tissue at risk and how much tissue is at risk?
4. Is there a vessel occlusion and where is it?
5. Is an intracerebral haemorrhage (ICH) or another underlying, non-ischaemic disease present?

Presently, the decision to initiate intravenous rt-PA treatment is based on clinical findings and CT scanning. The reported diagnostic yield of CT within 3 hours after symptom onset does not adequately meet these criteria.[24] The advent of new magnetic resonance imaging (MRI) techniques, such as perfusion- (PWI) and diffusion- (DWI) weighted imaging, has revolutionized diagnostic imaging in stroke.[71–76] DWI may delineate infarcted brain tissue in less than 1 hour after symptom onset, probably within minutes,[77] although there is increasing evidence that in the very early stage of stroke there may be reversible DWI changes,[78,79] while PWI defines the area of cerebral hypoperfusion. The absolute volume difference or ratio of PWI and DWI reveals the ischaemic tissue potentially at risk of irreversible infarction.[80,81] Magnetic resonance angiography (MRA) can reliably assess the cerebral vessel status.[82] Stroke MRI further allows a definitive diagnosis of ICH within the first hour of stroke,[83–85] and possibly also that of subarachnoid haemorrhage.[86] Several studies have reported early findings of stroke MRI within the first 6 to 12 hours, demonstrating the feasibility and practicality of this method in the setting of acute stroke and thrombolytic therapy.[72,75,80,87–91] In essence, the presence of a vessel occlusion according to MRA is associated with a PWI/DWI mismatch, the stroke MRI setting that defines the ideal candidate for thrombolysis.[89,92] Early recanalization achieved by thrombolysis results in significantly smaller infarcts and a significantly better clinical outcome.[79,80,89,91,93] Although presently limited by low availability, the utility of stroke MRI is likely to lie in the early identification of those patients in whom outcome and final infarct size, ultimately the patient's fate, have not yet been determined. Furthermore, cost-effectiveness is likely, as there is no need for CT or Doppler ultrasound in the hyperacute stage of stroke. With an increasing distribution and 'around the clock' availability of stroke MRI, the identification of patients more suitable for thrombolytic therapy, and those who are not, may lead to an increased benefit and a reduction in complications in patients receiving thrombolytic therapy.[89] Furthermore, the rather strictly defined therapeutic window may be qualified and individualized according to the findings in each individual patient.

Conclusion, recommendations and future prospects

Overall, thrombolysis with 0.9 mg/kg rt-PA for acute ischaemic stroke within 6 hours leads to a clinically significant effect in favour of treated patients but is associated with an excess rate of symptomatic intracerebral haemorrhage (ICH), which does, however, not take effect on mortality. Intravenous rt-PA (0.9 mg/kg; maximum of 90 mg) is therefore the recommended treatment within 3 hours after stroke symptom onset. The benefit from the use of intravenous rt-PA for acute ischaemic stroke beyond 3 h from onset of symptoms is lower, but definitely present in selected patients. Also, the European Stroke Initiative (EUSI) recommendations state that thrombolytic therapy is the treatment of choice within 3 hours and in selected patients up to 6 hours after stroke onset.[94] Intravenous rt-PA is not recommended when the time of onset of stroke cannot be ascertained reliably. Thrombolytic therapy should be peformed in centres experienced in the procedure. Intravenous administration of streptokinase for acute ischaemic stroke is dangerous and contraindicated. Data on the efficacy of other intravenously administered thrombolytic drugs are not available.

Intra-arterial thrombolysis with recombinant pro-urokinase (rpro-UK) is safe and effective within 6 hours after stroke onset, leading to a significantly higher rate of functional independence, also in patients with more severe baseline stroke symptoms. For vertebrobasilar artery thrombosis, intra-arterial thrombolysis, although not proven in randomized trials, if successful, may dramatically reduce mortality and disability, and therefore is the therapy of choice within 6 hours but eventually up to 12 hours after symptom onset. Improvements in early diagnostic evaluation of patients, particularly in magnetic resonance imaging (MRI) techniques, allow a better patient selection and possibly a qualification of the presently rigid therapeutic time frame.

At present, thrombolytic therapy is still underutilized. Among the major problems are that relatively few candidates meet the clinical and time criteria. Educating the general public to regard stroke as a treatable emergency and training emergency caregivers in the use of thrombolysis may decrease these problems. Health care institutions should be made aware of the potential in long-term cost savings, once stroke management is optimized and thrombolysis is more widely available. Patients and their relatives should be informed not only about the hazards of thrombolytic therapy but also about its potential benefit and thus the risk of *not* being treated.

References

1. WHO Task Force. Stroke–1989. Recommendations on stroke prevention, diagnosis, and therapy. Report of the WHO Task Force on Stroke and other Cerebrovascular Disorders. Stroke 1989; **20**:1407–31.

2. Hacke W, Steiner T, Schwab S. Critical management of the acute stroke: medical and surgical therapy. In: Batjer HH, Caplan LR, Freiberg L, Greenlee RG, Jr, Kopitnik TH, Jr, Young WL, eds, Cerebrovascular disease, 1st edn. (Lippincott-Raven: Hagerstown, Maryland, 1996) 523–33.

3. The GUSTO Angiographic investigators. The effects of tissue plasminogen activator, streptokinase or both on coronary artery patency, ventricular function, and survival after acute myocardial infarction. N Engl J Med 1993; **329**:1615–22.

4. Astrup J, Siesjö B, Symon L. Thresholds in cerebral ischemia—the ischemic penumbra. Stroke 1981; **12**:723–5.

5. Hacke W, Stingele R, Steiner T, Schuchardt V, Schwab S. Critical care of acute ischemic stroke. Intens Care Med 1995; **21**:856–62.

6. Hacke W, Willig V, Steiner T. Update on thrombolytic therapy in ischemic stroke. Fibrin Proteol 1997; **11**(suppl 2):1–4.

7. National Institute of Neurological Disorders and Stroke rt-PA Stroke Study Group. Tissue plasminogen activator for acute ischemic stroke. N Engl J Med 1995; **333**:1581–7.

8. Scandinavian Stroke Study Group. Multicenter trial of hemodilution in ischemic stroke. Stroke 1985; **16**:885–90.

9. Hacke W, Kaste M, Fieschi C et al. Intravenous thrombolysis with recombinant tissue plasminogen activator for acute hemispheric stroke. The European Cooperative Acute Stroke Study. JAMA 1995; **274**:1017–25.

10. Tillet WS, Garner RL. The fibrinolytic activity of hemolytic streptococci. J Exp Med 1933; **58**:485–502.

11. Meyer JS, Gilroy J, Barnhart MI, Johnson JF. Therapeutic thrombolysis in cerebral thromboembolism. Neurology 1963; **13**:927–37.

12. Abe T, Kazama M, Naito I. Clinical evaluation for efficacy of tissue cultured urokinase (TCUK) on cerebral thrombosis by means of multi-centre double blind study [Translated from Japanese]. Blood-Vessel 1981; **12**:321–41.

13. Atarashi J, Ohtomo E, Araki G, Itoh E, Togi H, Matsuda T. Clinical utility of urokinase in the treatment of acute stage cerebral thrombosis: multi-center double blind study in comparison with placebo [Translated from Japanese]. Clin Eval 1985; **13**:659–709.

14. Ohtomo E, Araki G, Itoh E, Toghi H, Matsuda T, Atarashi J. Clinical efficacy of urokinase in the treatment of cerebral thrombosis. Multi-center double blind study in comparison with placebo [Translated from Japanese]. Clin Eval 1985; **15**:711–31.

15. Haley EC, Jr, Brott TG, Sheppard GL et al. Pilot randomized trial of tissue plasminogen activator in acute ischemic stroke. The TPA Bridging Study Group. Stroke 1993; **24**:1000–4.

16. Mori E, Yoneda Y, Tabuchi M et al. Intravenous recombinant tissue plasminogen activator in acute carotid artery territory stroke. Neurology 1992; **42**:976–82.

17. Yamaguchi T, Hayakawa T, Kiuchi H, Japanese Thrombolysis Study Group. Intravenous tissue plasminogen activator ameliorates the outcome of hyperacute embolic stroke. Cerebrovasc Dis 1993; **3**:269–72.

18. Morris AD, Ritchie C, Grosset DG, Adams FG, Lees KR. A pilot study of streptokinase for acute cerebral infarction. QJM 1995; **88**:727–31.

19. The Multicentre Acute Stroke Trial–Italy (MAST-I) Group. Randomised controlled trial of streptokinase, aspirin, and combination of both in treatment of acute ischaemic stroke. Lancet 1995; **346**:1509–14.

20. Multicenter Acute Stroke Trial–Europe Study Group. Thrombolytic therapy with streptokinase in acute ischemic stroke. N Engl J Med 1996; **335**:145–50.

21. Donnan GA, Davis SM, Chambers BR et al. Streptokinase for acute ischemic stroke with relationship to time of administration: Australian Streptokinase (ASK) Trial Study Group. JAMA 1996; **276**:961–6.

22. Cornu C, Boutitie F, Candelise L et al. Streptokinase in acute ischemic stroke: an individual patient data meta-analysis: The Thrombolysis in Acute Stroke Pooling Project. Stroke 2000; **31**:1555–60.

23. Wardlaw JM, del Zoppo G, Yamaguchi T. Thrombolysis for acute ischaemic stroke (Cochrane Review). Cochrane Database Syst Rev 2000; issue 3.

24. Hacke W, Kaste M, Fieschi C et al. Randomised double-blind placebo-controlled trial of thrombolytic therapy with intravenous alteplase in acute ischaemic stroke (ECASS II). Lancet 1998; **352**:1245–51.

25. Clark WM, Wissman S, Albers GW, Jhamandas JH, Madden KP, Hamilton S. Recombinant tissue-type plasminogen activator (Alteplase) for ischemic stroke 3 to 5 hours after symptom onset. The ATLANTIS Study: a randomized controlled trial. Alteplase Thrombolysis for Acute Noninterventional Therapy in Ischemic Stroke. JAMA 1999; **282**:2019–26.

26. von Kummer R, Meyding-Lamade U, Forsting M et al. Sensitivity and prognostic value of early CT in occlusion of the middle cerebral artery trunk. Am J Neuroradiol 1994; **15**:9–15.

27. von Kummer R, Nolte PN, Schnittger H, Thron A, Ringelstein EB. Detectability of cerebral hemisphere ischaemic infarcts by CT within 6 h of stroke. Neuroradiology 1996; **38**:31–3.

28. von Kummer R, Allen KL, Holle R et al. Acute stroke: usefulness of early CT findings before thrombolytic therapy. Radiology 1997; **205**:327–33.

29. von Kummer R. Effect of training in reading CT scans on patient selection for ECASS II. Neurology 1998; **51** (suppl 3): S50–2.

30. Steiner T, Bluhmki E, Kaste M et al. The ECASS 3-hour cohort. Secondary analysis of ECASS data by time stratification. Cerebrovasc Dis 1998; **8**:198–203.

31. Hacke W, Brott T, Caplan L et al. Thrombolysis in acute ischemic

stroke: controlled trials and clinical experience. Neurology 1999; **53**:S3–14.

32. Wardlaw JM, Sandercock PA, Warlow CP, Lindley RI. Trials of thrombolysis in acute ischemic stroke: does the choice of primary outcome measure really matter? Stroke 2000; **31**:1133–5.

33. Grond M, Stenzel C, Schmulling S et al. Early intravenous thrombolysis for acute ischemic stroke in a community-based approach. Stroke 1998; **29**:1544–9.

34. Schmulling S, Grond M, Rudolf J, Heiss WD. One-year follow-up in acute stroke patients treated with rtPA in clinical routine. Stroke 2000; **31**:1552–4.

35. Chiu D, Krieger D, Villar-Cordova C et al. Intravenous tissue plasminogen activator for acute ischemic stroke—feasibility, safety and efficacy in the first year of clinical practice. Stroke 1998; **29**:18–22.

36. Albers GW, Bates VE, Clark WM, Bell R, Verro P, Hamilton SA. Intravenous tissue-type plasminogen activator for treatment of acute stroke: the Standard Treatment with Alteplase to Reverse Stroke (STARS) study. JAMA 2000; **283**:1145–50.

37. Katzan IL, Furlan AJ, Lloyd LE et al. Use of tissue-type plasminogen activator for acute ischemic stroke: the Cleveland area experience. JAMA 2000; **283**:1151–8.

38. TIMI Study Group. The Thrombolysis in Myocardial Infarction (TIMI) trial. Phase I findings. N Engl J Med 1985; **312**:932–6.

39. Barnwell SL, Clark WM, Nguyen TT, O'Neill OR, Wynn ML, Coull BM. Safety and efficacy of delayed intraarterial urokinase therapy with mechanical clot disruption for thromboembolic stroke. Am J Neuroradiol 1994; **15**:1817–22.

40. Ezura M, Kagawa S. Selective and superselective infusion of urokinase for embolic stroke. Surg Neurol 1992; **38**:353–8.

41. Gruber A, Nasel C, Lang W, Kitzmuller E, Bavinzski G, Czech T. Intra-arterial thrombolysis for the treatment of perioperative childhood cardioembolic stroke. Neurology 2000; **54**:1684–6.

42. Higashida RT, Halbach VV, Barnwell SL, Dowd CF, Hieshima GB. Thrombolytic therapy in acute stroke. J Endovasc Surg 1994; **1**:4–15.

43. Higashida RT, Halbach VV, Tsai FY, Dowd CF, Hieshima GB. Interventional neurovascular techniques for cerebral revascularization in the treatment of stroke. Am J Roentgenol 1994; **163**:793–800.

44. Jungreis CA, Wechsler LR, Horton JA. Intracranial thrombolysis via a catheter embedded in the clot. Stroke 1989; **20**:1578–80.

45. Mori E, Tabuchi M, Yoshida T, Yamadori A. Intracarotid urokinase with thromboembolic occlusion of the middle cerebral artery. Stroke 1988; **19**:802–12.

46. Sasaki O, Takeuchi S, Koike T, Koizumi T, Tanaka R. Fibrinolytic therapy for acute embolic stroke: intravenous, intracarotid, and intra-arterial local approaches. Neurosurgery 1995; **36**:246–52.

47. Theron J, Courtheoux P, Casasco A et al. Local intraarterial fibrinolysis in the carotid territory. Am J Neuroradiol 1989; **10**:753–65.

48. Ueda T, Sakaki S, Kumon Y, Ohta S. Multivariable analysis of predictive factors related to outcome at 6 months after intra-arterial

thrombolysis for acute ischemic stroke. Stroke 1999; **30**:2360–5.

49. Ueda T, Sakaki S, Yuh WT, Nochide I, Ohta S. Outcome in acute stroke with successful intra-arterial thrombolysis and predictive value of initial single-photon emission-computed tomography. J Cereb Blood Flow Metab 1999; **19**:99–108.

50. del Zoppo GJ, Ferbert A, Otis S et al. Local intra-arterial fibri-nolytic therapy in acute carotid territory stroke. A pilot study. Stroke 1988; **19**:307–13.

51. Jansen O, von Kummer R, Forsting M, Hacke W, Sartor K. Thrombolytic therapy in acute occlusion of the intracranial inter-nal carotid artery bifurcation. Am J Neuroradiol 1995; **16**:1977–86.

52. Zeumer H. Vascular recanalizing technique in interventional neuro-radiology. J Neurol 1985; **231**:287–94.

53. Zeumer H, Freitag HJ, Zanella F, Thie A, Arning C. Local intra-arte-rial fibrinolytic therapy in patients with stroke: urokinase versus recombinant tissue plasminogen activator (r-TPA). Neuroradiology 1993; **35**:159–62.

54. Lewandowski CA, Frankel M, Tomsick TA et al. Combined intravenous and intra-arterial r-TPA versus intra-arterial therapy of acute ischemic stroke: Emergency Management of Stroke (EMS) Bridging Trial. Stroke 1999; **30**:2598–605.

55. del Zoppo GJ, Higashida RT, Furlan AJ et al. PROACT: a phase II randomized trial of recombinant pro-urokinase by direct arterial delivery in acute middle cerebral artery stroke. Stroke 1998; **29**:4–11.

56. Furlan A, Higashida R, Wechsler L et al. Intra-arterial prourokinase

for acute ischemic stroke. The PROACT II study: a randomized controlled trial. Prolyse in Acute Cerebral Thromboembolism. JAMA 1999; **282**:2003–11.

57. Brandt T, von Kummer R, Muller Kuppers M, Hacke W. Thrombolytic therapy of acute basilar artery occlusion. Variables affecting recanalization and outcome. Stroke 1996; **27**:875–81.

58. Hacke W, Zeumer H, Ferbert A, Brückmann H, del Zoppo G. Intraarterial thrombolytic therapy improves outcome in patients with acute vertebrobasilar occlu-sive disease. Stroke 1988; **19**:1216–22.

59. Brandt T, Knauth M, Wildermuth S et al. CT angiography and Doppler sonography for emer-gency assessment in acute basilar artery ischemia. Stroke 1999; **30**:606–12.

60. Bozzao L, Bastianello S, Fantozzi LM, Angeloni U, Argentino C, Fieschi C. Correlation of angio-graphic and sequential CT find-ings in patients with evolving cerebral infarction. Am J Neuro-radiol 1989; **10**:1215–22.

61. Truwit CL, Barkovich AJ, Gean-Marton A, Hibri N, Norman D. Loss of the insular ribbon: another early CT sign of acute middle cerebral artery infarction. Radiology 1990; **176**:801–6.

62. Horowitz SH, Zito JL, Donnarumma R, Patel M, Alvir J. Computed tomographic-angio-graphic findings within the first five hours of cerebral in-farction. Stroke 1991; **22**:1245–53.

63. Tomsick TA, Brott TG, Chambers AA et al. Hyperdense middle cerebral artery sign on CT: efficacy in detecting middle cerebral artery thrombosis. Am J Neuroradiol 1990; **11**:473–7.

64. Tomsick T, Brott T, Barsan W et al. Prognostic value of the hyperdense middle cerebral artery sign and stroke scale score before ultra early thrombolytic therapy. Am J Neuroradiol 1996; **17**:1–7.

65. Leys D, Pruvo JP, Godefroy O, Rondepierre P, Leclerc X. Prevalence and significance of hyperdense middle cerebral artery in acute stroke. Stroke 1992; **23**:317–24.

66. Bozzao L, Angeloni U, Bastianello S, Fantozzi LM, Pierallini A, Fieschi C. Early angiographic and CT findings in patients with hemorrhagic infarction in the distribution of the middle cerebral artery. Am J Neuroradiol 1991; **12**: 1115–21.

67. Schriger DL, Kalafut M, Starkman S, Krueger M, Saver JL. Cranial computed tomography interpretation in acute stroke: physician accuracy in determining eligibility for thrombolytic therapy. JAMA 1998; **279**:1293–7.

68. Knauth M, Kummer Rv, Jansen O, Haehnel S, Doerfler A, Sartor K. Potential of CT angiography in acute ischemic stroke. Am J Neuroradiol 1997; **18**:1001–10.

69. Doerfler A, Engelhorn T, von Kummer R et al. Are iodinated contrast agents detrimental in acute cerebral ischemia? An experimental study in rats. Radiology 1998; **206**:211–17.

70. Wildermuth S, Knauth M, Brandt T, Winter R, Sartor K, Hacke W. Role of CT angiography in patient selection for thrombolytic therapy in acute hemispheric stroke. Stroke 1998; **29**:935–8.

71. Sorensen AG, Buonanno FS, Gonzalez RG et al. Hyperacute stroke: evaluation with combined multisection diffusion-weighted and hemodynamically weighted echo-planar MR imaging. Radiology 1996; **199**:391–401.

72. Tong DC, Yenari MA, Albers GW, O'Brien M, Marks MP, Moseley ME. Correlation of perfusion- and diffusion-weighted MRI with NIHSS score in acute (< 6.5 hour) ischemic stroke. Neurology 1998; **50**:864–70.

73. Warach S, Dashe JF, Edelman RR. Clinical outcome in ischemic stroke predicted by early diffusion-weighted and perfusion magnetic resonance imaging: a preliminary analysis. J Cereb Blood Flow Metab 1996; **16**:53–9.

74. Warach S, Boska M, Welch KM. Pitfalls and potential of clinical diffusion-weighted MR imaging in acute stroke. Stroke 1997; **28**:481–2.

75. Barber PA, Darby DG, Desmond PM et al. Prediction of stroke outcome with echoplanar perfusion- and diffusion-weighted MRI. Neurology 1998; **51**:418–26.

76. Moseley ME, Wendland MF, Kucharczyk J. Magnetic resonance imaging of diffusion and perfusion. Top Magn Reson Imaging 1991; **3**:50–67.

77. Conturo TE, McKinstry RC, Aronovitz JA, Neil JJ. Diffusion MRI: precision, accuracy and flow effects. NMR Biomed 1995; **8**:307–32.

78. Kidwell CS, Alger JR, F Di Salle et al. Diffusion MRI in patients with transient ischemic attacks. Stroke 1999; **30**:1174–80.

79. Kidwell CS, Saver JL, Mattiello J et al. Thrombolytic reversal of acute human cerebral ischemic injury shown by diffusion/perfusion magnetic resonance imaging. Ann Neurol 2000; **47**: 462–9.

80. Jansen O, Schellinger PD, Fiebach JB, Hacke W, Sartor K. Early recanalization in acute

ischemic stroke saves tissue at risk defined by MRI. Lancet 1999; **353**:2036–7.

81. Schlaug G, Benfield A, Baird AE et al. The ischemic penumbra: operationally defined by diffusion and perfusion MRI. Neurology 1999; **53**:1528–37.

82. Jansen O, Heiland S, Schellinger P. Neuroradiological diagnosis in acute ischemic stroke. Value of modern techniques. Nervenarzt 1998; **69**:465–71.

83. Linfante I, Llinas RH, Caplan LR, Warach S. MRI features of intracerebral hemorrhage within 2 hours from symptom onset. Stroke 1999; **30**:2263–7.

84. Patel MR, Edelman RR, Warach S. Detection of hyperacute primary intraparenchymal hemorrhage by magnetic resonance imaging. Stroke 1996; **27**:2321–4.

85. Schellinger PD, Jansen O, Fiebach JB, Hacke W, Sartor K. A standardized MRI stroke protocol: comparison with CT in hyperacute intracerebral hemorrhage. Stroke 1999; **30**:765–8.

86. Wiesmann M, Mayer T, Yousri I et al. Comparison of FLAIR and fast spin-echo MR imaging at 1.5T for detection of acute subarachnoid hemorrhage. Joint Annual Meeting of the American Society of Neuroradiology, 22–28 May, San Diego, CA, 1999.

87. Baird AE, Warach S. Imaging developing brain infarction. Curr Opin Neurol 1999; **12**:65–71.

88. Beaulieu C, de Crespigny A, Tong DC, Moseley ME, Albers GW, Marks MP. Longitudinal magnetic resonance imaging study of perfusion and diffusion in stroke: evolution of lesion volume and correlation with clinical outcome. Ann Neurol 1999; **46**:568–78.

89. Schellinger PD, Jansen O, Fiebach JB et al. Monitoring intravenous recombinant tissue plasminogen activator thrombolysis for acute ischemic stroke with diffusion and perfusion MRI. Stroke 2000; **31**:1318–28.

90. Schellinger PD, Jansen O, Fiebach JB et al. Feasibility and practicality of MR imaging of stroke in the management of hyperacute cerebral ischemia. Am J Neuroradiol 2000; **21**:1184–9.

91. Schellinger PD, Fiebach JB, Jansen O et al. Stroke magnetic resonance imaging within 6 hours after onset of hyperacute cerebral ischemia. Ann Neurol 2001; **49**:460–9.

92. Rordorf G, Koroshetz WJ, Copen WA et al. Regional ischemia and ischemic injury in patients with acute middle cerebral artery stroke as defined by early diffusion-weighted and perfusion-weighted MRI. Stroke 1998; **49**:939–43.

93. Marks MP, Tong D, Beaulieu C, Albers G, de Crespigny A, Moseley ME. Evaluation of early reperfusion and IV rt-PA therapy using diffusion- and perfusion-weighted MRI. Neurology 1999; **52**:1792–8.

94. European Stroke Initiative. Recommendations for stroke management. Cerebrovasc Dis 2000; **10**(suppl 3):1–34.

Index

abciximab 105–7
ACE inhibitors 78–9
acute myocardial infarction (AMI)
  ACE inhibitors 78–9
  adenosine 85–6
  adjunctive therapy, anticoagulants 63–73
  aspirin 23–4
  benefits, thrombolysis 23
  beta blockers 76–8
  calcium 88
  calcium channel blockers 79–82
  cardiogenic shock 104–5
  clinical guidelines 32–4, 33
  clinical opportunities 20
  complement inhibition 88
  GIK 86
  heparin 63–7
  lipid lowering drugs 84–5
  LMWHs 63–7, 67
  magnesium 82–3
  neutrophils 87
  nitrates 84
  oxygen free radicals 88
  patient selection, thrombolytic therapy 31–4
  pharmacological interventions 75–95
  platelets 87
  principles, fibrinolytic therapy 19–38
  problems with thrombolytics 29–31
  reperfusion 75–6
  restoring vessel patency 20–2
  risks, thrombolysis 23
  thrombolysis, clinical trials 22–8
  see also myocardial infarction
adenosine, AMI 85–6
adjunctive therapy, anticoagulants 63–73, 67, 68
alteplase (rt-PA)
  adjuvants 63–6, 65
  pharmacodynamics 9–10
  pharmacology 10
  physicochemical properties 1–5
  regimens 33
  structure 4, 25
  thrombolytic activation, plasminogen 21
AMI see acute myocardial infarction
anaphylaxis, thrombolytic agents problem 29
angioplasty
  balloon 105–7, 106
  facilitated 52–3
  vs fibrinolytic therapy 97–100, 98, 99, 100,
    101, 127–8
  primary 50–2
  vs stenting 105–7
angiotensin-converting enzyme (ACE) inhibitors

AMI 78–9
  mechanisms of action 78
anistreplase (APSAC)
  pharmacodynamics 12
  pharmacology 10
  physicochemical properties 5–6
  thrombolytic activation, plasminogen 21
anticoagulants
  adjunctive therapy 63–73
  oral 66–70, 68
antiplatelet therapy 39–61
  MI, acute phase 42–53
  MI, chronic phase 53–7
  pathogenesis 39–42
antithrombin therapy, fibrinolysis 63–6
APSAC see anistreplase
aspirin
  adjuvants 66–70, 68
  AMI 23–4
  MI, acute phase 42–4, 43
  MI, chronic phase 53–5

balloon angioplasty, vs stenting 105–7, 106
beta blockers
  AMI 76–8
  mechanisms of action 76–7
  thrombolytic therapy combination 77–8
bleeding, thrombolytic agents problem 29
bolus thrombolytics 24–7
  summary 27

calcium, AMI 88
calcium channel blockers
  AMI 79–82
  diltiazem 81
  nifedipine 80–1
  verapamil 82
cardiogenic shock, AMI 104–5
catheter-directed fibrinolytic therapy, DVT
  133–6
clinical guidelines, AMI 32–4, 33
clinical trials
  antithrombin therapy, fibrinolysis 63–6
  intra-arterial thrombolysis 163–5
  ischaemic stroke 153–60
  MI, acute phase 42–53
  MI, chronic phase 53–7
  pre-hospital fibrinolytic therapy 116–20, 117,
    119
  pre-hospital vs in-hospital fibrinolysis 116–20,
    117, 119, 125, 126
  streptokinase 23–4
  thrombolysis 22–8

clopidogrel
   MI, acute phase 44
   MI, chronic phase 55–6
complement inhibition, AMI 88
computed tomography (CT), ischaemic stroke
   165–7
contraindications, thrombolysis 33
CT see computed tomography
cyclooxygenase, aspirin 42–4, 43

dalteparin, adjuvant 63–6, 65
deep vein thrombosis (DVT) 131–6
   anticoagulant therapy 132–6
   fibrinolytic therapy 132–6
   heparin 132–6, 134
   streptokinase 134
   vitamin K antagonists 132–6
delay, treatment see treatment delay
diagnostic imaging, ischaemic stroke 165–7
diltiazem, AMI 81
Dutch experience, pre-hospital fibrinolytic
   therapy 124–6
DVT see deep vein thrombosis

enoxaparin, adjuvant 63–6, 65, 67

facilitated angioplasty 52–3
fibrinolytic therapy, vs angioplasty 97–100, 98,
   99, 100, 101, 127–8

GIK see glucose-insulin-potassium
glucose-insulin-potassium (GIK), AMI 86
GP IIb/IIIa antagonists
   MI, acute phase 44–53
   MI, chronic phase 56–7

heparin
   AMI 63–7
   DVT 132–6, 134
   PE 137, 139, 141–3

indications, thrombolysis 33
intra-arterial thrombolysis
   ischaemic stroke 163–5
   PROACT trials 163–5
intravenous thrombolysis, ischaemic stroke
   152–62
ischaemic stroke 153–73
   ATLANTIS trial 155
   conclusion 167
   CT 165–7
   diagnostic imaging 165–7
   ECASS trials 153–4, 156–60
   future prospects 167
   intra-arterial thrombolysis 163–5
   intravenous thrombolysis 152–62
   meta-analyses 155–61
   NINDS trial 153, 156–60
   patient assessment, initial 151–2
   recommendations 167
   rt-PA 153
   streptokinase 152

lanoteplase (n-PA)
   pharmacodynamics 9–11
   pharmacology 10
   physicochemical properties 4–5

structure 4, 25
treatment improvement 26
lipid lowering drugs, AMI 84–5
low molecular weight heparins (LMWHs)
   AMI 63–7, 67
   DVT 132–6
   see also heparin

magnesium, AMI 82–3
mechanisms of action
   ACE inhibitors 78
   beta blockers 76–7
   thrombolytic agents 6–8
MI see myocardial infarction
microvascular function, reperfusion 86–7
microvascular perfusion, and vessel patency
   27–8
monteplase
   pharmacodynamics 10–11
   pharmacology 10
   physicochemical properties 4–5
   structure 4
myocardial infarction (MI)
   antiplatelet therapy, acute phase 42–53
   antiplatelet therapy, chronic phase 53–7
   oral anticoagulation 66–70, 68
   see also acute myocardial infarction

neutrophils, AMI 87
nifedipine, AMI 80–1
nitrates, AMI 84
'no reflow phenomenon' 28

oral anticoagulation, MI 66–70, 68
oxygen free radicals, AMI 88

pamiteplase
   pharmacology 10
   structure 4
patency see vessel patency
pathogenesis, antiplatelet therapy 39–42
patient selection, thrombolytic therapy 31–4
PE see pulmonary embolism
pentasaccharide, adjuvant 63–6, 65
percutaneous coronary intervention, ST-segment
   elevation 97–110
percutaneous transluminal coronary angioplasty
   (PTCA) 100–4, 101, 102
pharmacodynamics, thrombolytic agents 8–13
pharmacological interventions, AMI 75–95
pharmacology, thrombolytic agents 1–18
physicochemical properties, thrombolytic agents
   1–6
plasmin, formation 2
plasminogen
   activation 2
   thrombolytic activation 21
platelet activation 40–2, 41
platelet aggregation 40–2, 41
platelets, AMI 87
practical guidelines, PE 145–6
pre-hospital fibrinolytic therapy 111–30
   benefits 120–3
   clinical trials 116–20, 117, 119
   Dutch experience 124–6
   pre-hospital triage 113–16
   risks 120–3

primary angioplasty 50–2
prothrombotic state, increased 44–7, *46*
PTCA *see* percutaneous transluminal coronary
   angioplasty
pulmonary embolism (PE) 136–45
   clinical outcomes 138–40
   dose regimen 144–5
   fibrinolytic therapy 137–46
   heparin 137, *139*, *141–3*
   massive 144
   practical guidelines 145–6
   right ventricular dysfunction 144
   safety bleedings 140
   vitamin K antagonists 137

reperfusion
   AMI 75–6
   microvascular function 86–7
reteplase (r-PA)
   mechanisms of action 7
   pharmacodynamics 9–10
   pharmacology *10*
   physicochemical properties 3–5
   regimens *33*
   structure *4*, *25*
   thrombolytic activation, plasminogen *21*
   treatment improvement 24–6
ridogrel, MI, acute phase 44
right ventricular dysfunction, PE 144
rt-PA *see* alteplase

safety bleedings, PE 140
Sak *see* staphylokinase
saruplase, pharmacology *10*
ST-segment elevation, percutaneous coronary
   intervention 97–110
staphylokinase (Sak)
   mechanisms of action 8
   pharmacodynamics 12–13
   pharmacology *10*
   physicochemical properties 6
statins, AMI 84–5
stenting, vs balloon angioplasty 105–7, *106*
streptokinase
   clinical trials 23–4
   DVT *134*
   ischaemic stroke 152
   mechanisms of action 7–8
   pharmacodynamics 11–12
   pharmacology *10*
   physicochemical properties 5–6
   regimens *33*
   thrombolytic activation, plasminogen *21*
stroke
   thrombolytic agents problem 29
   see also ischaemic stroke

t-PA
   adjuvants 63–6, *65*
   mechanisms of action 6–7
   pharmacodynamics 8–11
   physicochemical properties 1–5
   primary structure *3*
TAFI *see* Thrombin Activatable Fibrinolysis
   Inhibitor
tenecteplase (TNK-rt-PA)
   mechanisms of action 7
   pharmacology *10*
   physicochemical properties 4–5
   regimens *33*
   structure *4*, *25*
   thrombolytic activation, plasminogen *21*
   treatment improvement 26–7
Thrombin Activatable Fibrinolysis Inhibitor (TAFI)
   45
thrombolysis
   after 31
   clinical trials 22–8
   contraindications *33*
   failed *30*, 30
   indications *33*
   treatment schedules 32–4, *33*
thrombolytic agents
   mechanisms of action 6–8
   pharmacodynamics 8–13
   pharmacology 1–18
   physicochemical properties 1–6
   problems 29–31
thrombolytic therapy
   beta blockers combination 77–8
   patient selection 31–4
ticlopidine, MI, acute phase 44
treatment delay 31–2, *32*, 111–16, *113*, *114*, *115*
   clinical practice 113–16
treatment schedules 32–4, *33*
trials *see* clinical trials

u-PA moieties
   mechanisms of action 7
   pharmacodynamics 11
   physicochemical properties 5

venous thromboembolism 131–49
   DVT 131–6
   PE 136–45
verapamil, AMI 82
vessel patency
   and microvascular perfusion 27–8
   restoring 20–2
vitamin K antagonists
   DVT 132–6
   PE 137
von Willebrand's factor (vWF) 40